staying power

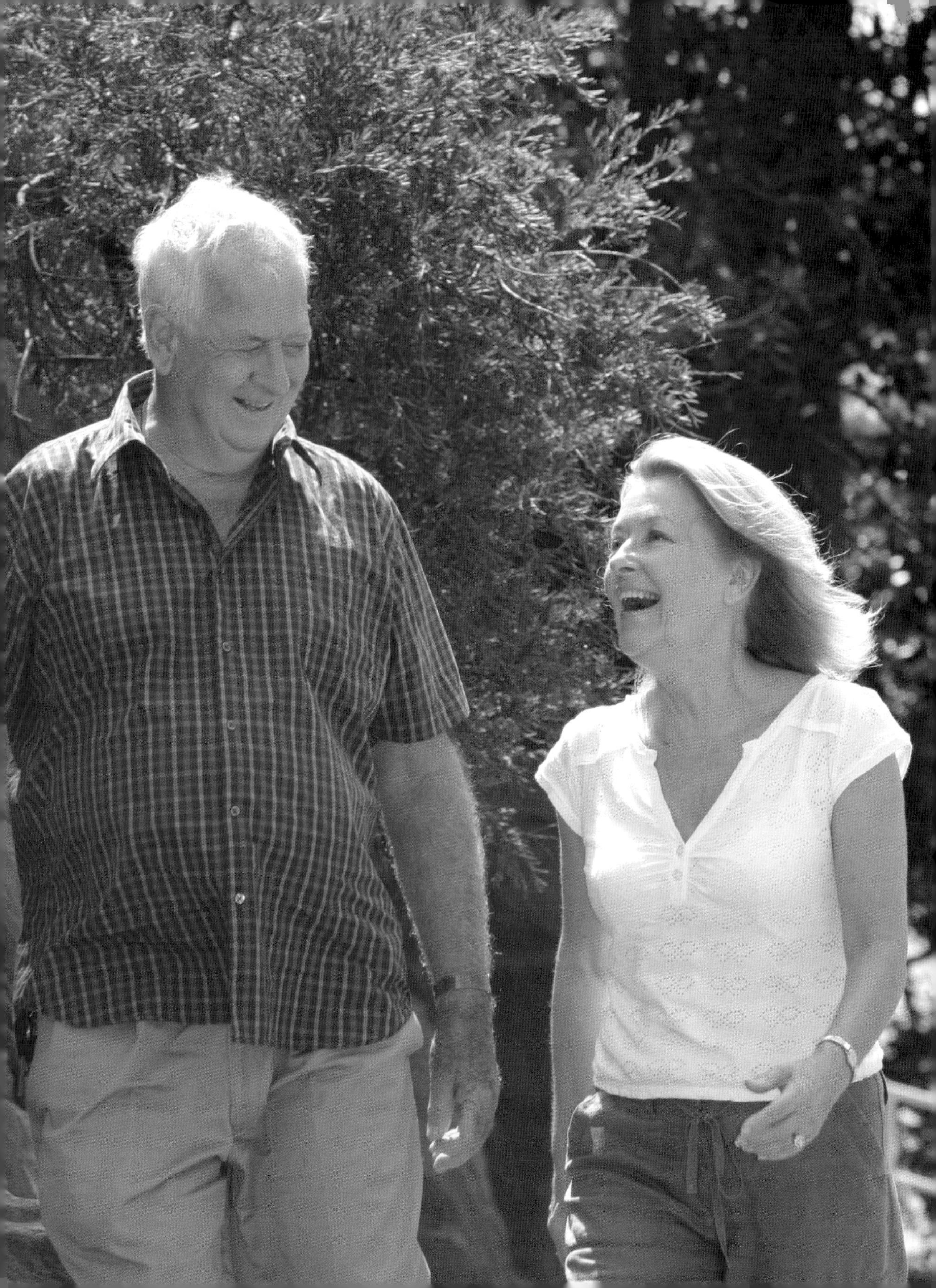

staying power

tips and tools to keep you on your feet

Lindy Clemson and
Megan Swann-Williams

Every effort has been made in compiling this book to provide accurate and up-to-date information with accepted standards and practice at the time of publication. Nevertheless, the authors and publisher can make no warranties that the information contained herein is totally free of error, not least because clinical standards are constantly changing through research and regulation. The authors and publisher therefore disclaim all liability for direct or consequential damages resulting from the use of material contained in this book.

Limelight Press Pty Ltd
Unit 15, 6 Thames Street
Balmain NSW 2041
ABN 80 095 617 897

Published by Limelight Press Pty Ltd 2006

National Library of Australia
Cataloguing-in-Publication data:

Clemson, Lindy.
Staying power : tips and tools to keep you on your feet.

Includes index.
ISBN 0 9775361 0 6.

1. Falls (Accidents) in old age - Prevention - Handbooks, manuals, etc. 2. Accidents - Prevention - Handbooks, manuals, etc. I. Swann-Williams, Megan. II. Title.

613.60846

Photography by Kathy Carr, KTS Photographics
Designed by Avril Makula
Printed and bound by SNP-Leefung, China

contents

about this book

One of the intentions of this book is to support the Stepping On group program, acting as a reference aid for participants to help them maintain all that they have learnt. But if you haven't been to the group, don't worry.

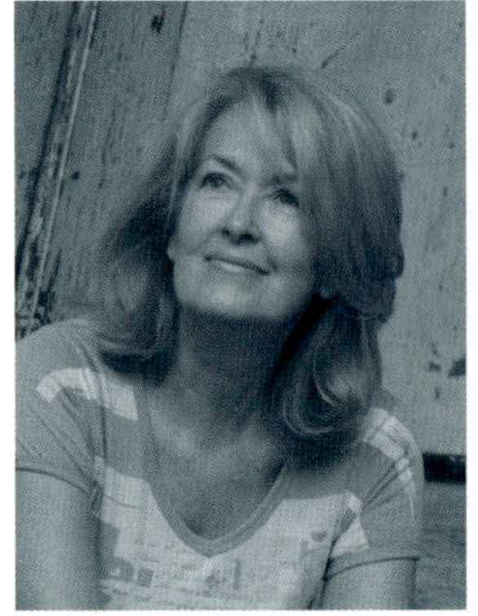

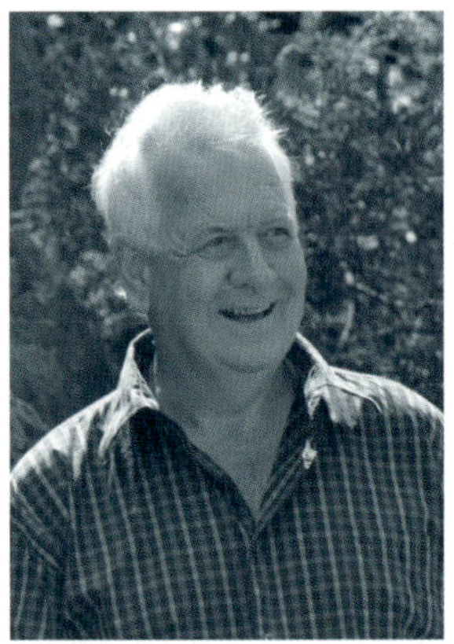

This book is primarily designed for those who are completely new to the concept of falls reduction. It serves as an introduction to the idea, a source of practical information on how to go about it, and a guide to overcoming the challenges you may face. By taking time to think about the points we raise, it will help you build self-awareness of your own falls risks and confidence in your mobility.

From time to time we will introduce you to people's stories to help illustrate points we are making. These stories have all come from real people who have attended the groups. They have shared their fall experiences, their fears as well as the fall prevention activities they have used. They have worked energetically and with commitment to reduce their risk of falling, strengthening their independent lifestyle and, in many cases, giving themselves a new outlook on their life.

In "Part 2: boosters and barriers to a safer life style" we address some possible barriers to your success. We look at issues such as ageist social myths about falls, a lack of confidence, unrealistic expectations and feedback from families and friends. We also suggest ways to combat these barriers. It is incredibly important to have a positive approach to falls reduction, so we will be focusing on what you are able to do when facing these challenges, rather than just pointing out the difficulties you may face. Part 2 provides a positive,

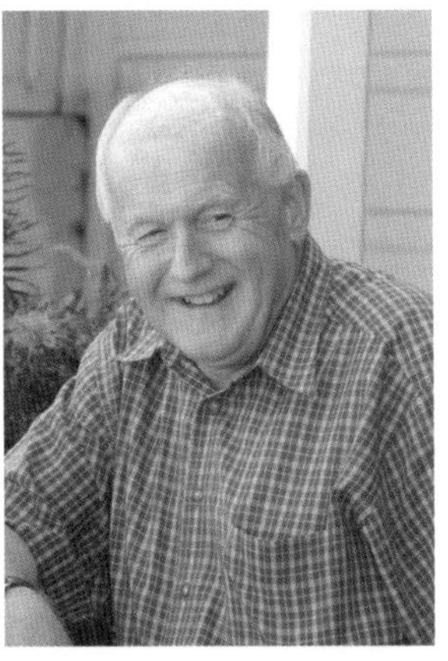

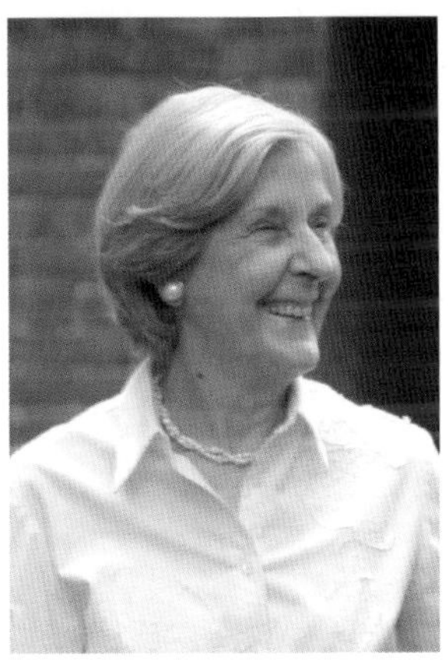

This information will guide you towards safety, confidence and independence.

constructive mental framework to help you get the most out of this book.

"Part 3: how to keep you on your feet" is the main thrust of the book. It covers three main falls reduction topics, each in its own section:

- Moving
- Feeling safe at home and in your community
- How to handle a changing body

Each of these topics focuses on one key aspect of falls reduction. Through these topics, we provide you with the explanations and opportunities that will enable you to identify your own falls risks and reduce the chances of them eventuating into the trauma of a fall. By using real-life examples, discussing the issues involved, suggesting practical solutions and strategies for implementing these solutions and explaining why they work, this information will guide you towards safety, confidence and independence.

Of course, if you want to get straight into the main topics, it is quite acceptable to skip Part 2. However if you have a question about a certain area or you need a reminder about something specific later on, just look up the relevant topic in the contents or index—the book is flexible enough to serve as either a reference source or a complete guidebook. It is a good idea to keep Part 2 in mind, however, just in case you come up against any barriers to your progress when you get further down the track, such as feeling unsure or reaching a stumbling block.

We show you tools and strategies that have been proven to work, but part of the effectiveness of these strategies is that they aren't just a list of rules. There is no pill anyone can give you that will help build your confidence and reduce the risk of falls; the challenges of falls reduction are yours and yours alone.

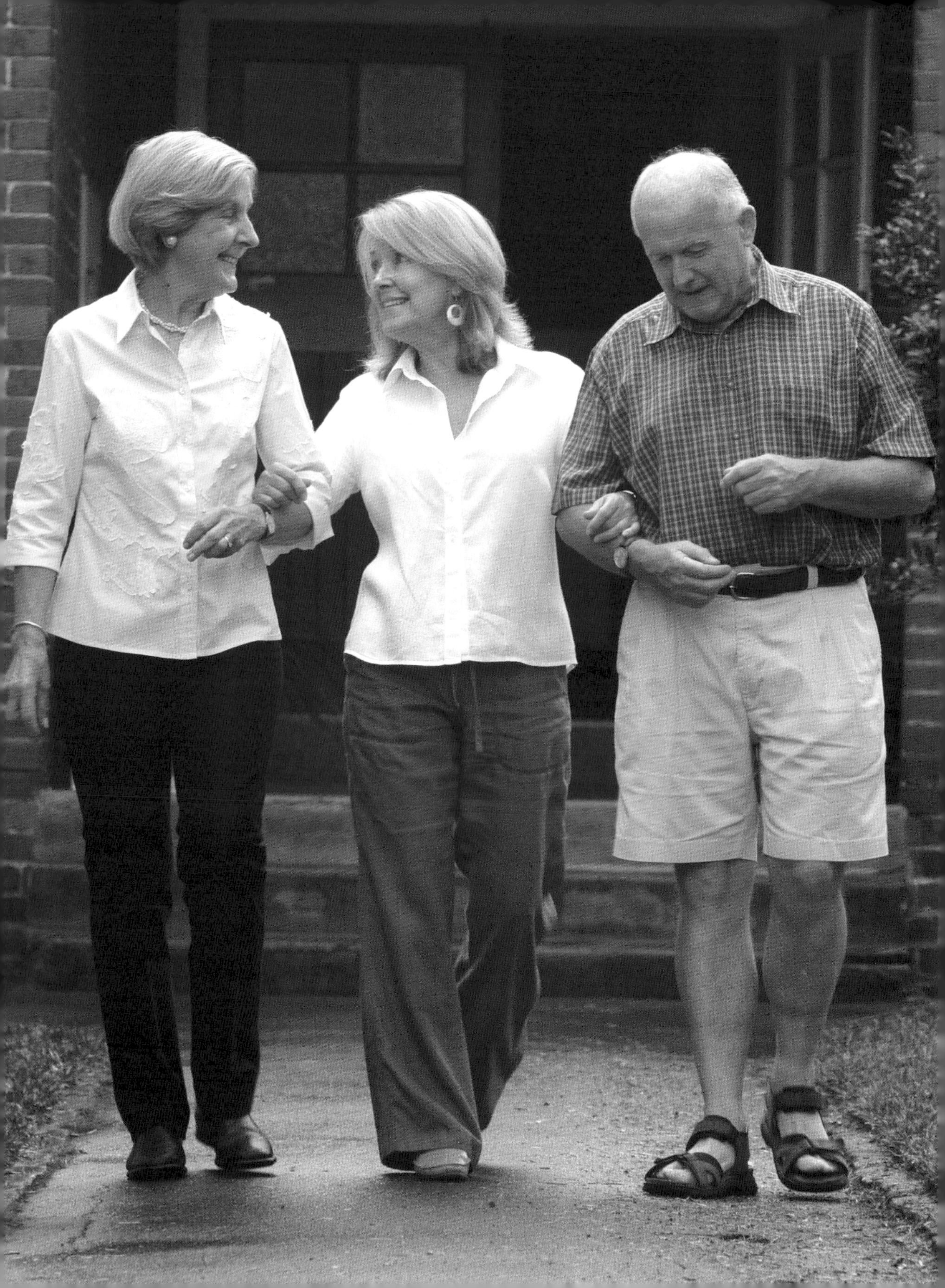

PART 1

staying on your feet

CHAPTER 1

coming to grips with falls

Having a fall gives anyone a shock. Falls can affect us all, no matter what age or level of fitness. They are not an inevitable consequence of growing older—you can do a lot to reduce your own risk of falling. It's simply a matter of employing a new way of thinking about a very old problem.

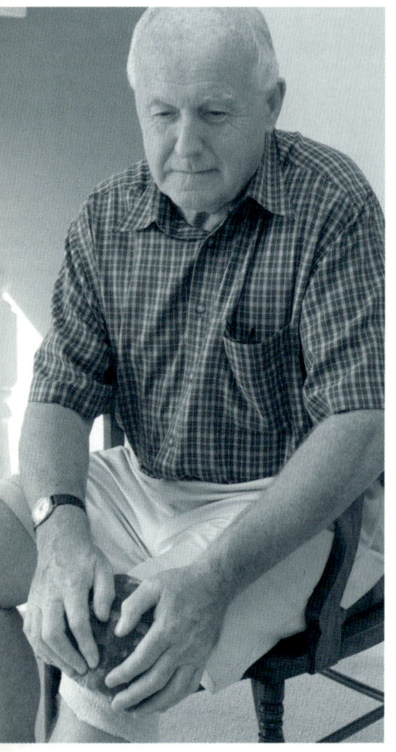

Your chances of having a fall increase as you get older

A fall presents a much higher risk if you are older. Not only is there more risk of physically damaging bone and tissue, and more chance of not fully recovering, you are actually at greater risk of having a fall in the first place.

When you are older, the after-effects of soft tissue injury or even a fracture that results from a fall can be far-reaching. In one year, a third of older people will have a fall. Of these, one in ten will have a major injury as a result.

The number of people who fall each year increases as you get older, so that by the age of ninety, over 40 per cent of us will experience at least one fall per year. Half of these people admit to being afraid of falling. One in three people who fall will be less active as a result, often restricting activities such as going out, shopping and housework.

A traumatising experience

A fall can be a frightening and traumatising experience. While some people do recover and move on, many people find the physical and psychological consequences devastating. People often lose their confidence and do less physical activity, which can lead to a downward spiral of incapacity. We have all heard stories of a fall leading to a person's loss of independence, to facing life in a nursing home and even, to death.

Research shows that people who have experienced one or more falls in a year can be far more motivated to change their behaviour and reduce their risk of falling. So chances are that you are reading this book because in the last couple of years you have already experienced the frightening consequences of a fall. You may have experienced falls indirectly through friends or family who have had a fall and related their story to you. Regardless of why, it's safe to say that you are reading this book because you actively want to reduce your falls risk.

Falls can affect us all, no matter what age or level of fitness.

Understanding falls and how to reduce them

Reducing falls for older people is a new and exciting area of research. While it is still a young field of study, we already know so much more than we ever did about why people fall, what the consequences can be, and most importantly, what we can do to try to prevent falls.

Facing the fall factors

Many factors influence your likelihood of falling. They can relate to your physical state, awareness of danger, personal attitude and general lifestyle. If you address these factors, your chance of having a fall can dramatically decrease, even when you are faced with an external obstacle, such as a slippery floor or a gutter. This approach to health comes under the banner of preventive medicine.

meet Joan

Joan was walking down the back outside steps of her daughter's house. She had just finished reading the paper, but had forgotten to take off her bifocals. She was wearing high heels and was recovering from the flu. The steps were wet, slippery and mossy, and her daughter's Burmese cats were milling at the bottom, wanting to finish their dinner. As Joan walked down the steps, she swayed, lost her balance and fell, fracturing her ankle.

Since this fall, Joan has never worn high heels again and she has lost her confidence to walk alone outside her house. She says that she no longer goes to line dancing and really misses meeting her friends afterwards for coffee. She has stopped many community activities, which is making her body slow down. She feels older and lonely.

COMMENT

Joan's lack of confidence led to her downward spiral. Because she was doing less, she became weaker, which made her even more vulnerable to falling.

Joan's potential to reduce her risk of falling is influenced by how confident she is to balance and to avoid falls. Being more aware of what made her fall and how to prevent it will also reduce her risk.

THINK A MOMENT

- What factors contributed to Joan's fall?
- What do you think Joan could have done to reduce her risk of falling and increase her confidence again?
- When you have finished reading this book, come back to Joan's story and make another list of causes and potential solutions for Joan.
- What barriers might Joan need to overcome to get control of her life again?

By reducing your chance of falling, you can live more confidently and remain independent. Having a positive, constructive and realistic attitude towards falls reduction will result in you being able to take control of your life.

The real success of the Stepping On program is due to the participants, who have reflected on the information, worked out what they needed to do and decided to take action.

The Stepping On program

The ideas in this book are based on a program we have developed called Stepping On. This community group-based program draws on the most up-to-date knowledge on falls and how to prevent them. It combines many varied but vital elements into one integrated approach for lessening the risk of falls.

The Stepping On groups meet at a central venue in the community, where the participants discuss their experiences of falls with each other under the guidance of a "group facilitator", who is a trained health professional. Via the facilitator, the group works through the various topic areas, discussing and practising useful strategies for overcoming the factors that contribute to falls.

The Stepping On program has been scientifically proven to work. Research findings have been translated into real life by combining different approaches that have evolved from these findings into one source. The program looks at a range of issues, from physical fitness to lifestyle choices, and explains how to overcome these personal risk factors.

But the real success of the program is due to the participants who have reflected on the information, worked out what they needed to do and decided to take action.

meet Vera

Vera had just woken up and was feeling a bit groggy from the sleeping tablets she took the night before. She shuffled into her old slippers and wandered out of the bedroom. She was feeling light-headed, which made it a bit tricky for her to go down the stairs, but she was thinking more about her breakfast than anything else.

When Vera got to the kitchen, she opened a cupboard above her head and reached up to grab her teapot. The blood rushed from her head and she suddenly felt faint. Vera staggered backwards, trying to regain her balance, but her ill-fitting slippers gave no support and as she stumbled, her feet slid out from under her. She tripped and fell, landing hard on her kitchen floor. Lying on her side in agonising pain, Vera was unable to get up. Then, with final determination, she managed to heave herself up just enough to pull the phone down, and she hastily dialled for an ambulance.

The whole experience was crushing. Apart from the embarrassment, she was in a lot of pain for weeks afterwards because she had fractured her hip bone when she fell. After the fall, Vera's hip never really felt strong again. When Vera finally returned home, she felt intimidated by even the simplest daily tasks. She felt powerless, as though she'd lost control of her life.

COMMENT

Comfortable home footwear is often in a state of disrepair with little support and worn, slippery soles. Vera's reliance on sleeping tablets, however, was the major contributor to her fall. A prescription for one night can turn into a prescription for life. Vera may well have been able to reduce her tablet dose. She may even have been able to manage her sleep problems in other ways.

THINK A MOMENT

- Vera blamed only her ill-fitting slippers as the cause of her fall and quite clearly they did contribute. But were they the only reason Vera fell?
- How could Vera be more aware of the side effects of her medication?
- How could Vera review her need for medication?

CHAPTER 2

the causes and cures of falls

As you get older, many changes can happen gradually so that you tend not to notice them. You can become less active, your bones can become more brittle, your muscles weaker, your balance less stable and your eyesight less clear. It happens so slowly over a number of years that it's hard to identify exactly what these changes are.

Usually, you just go about your life as you always have until one day the effects of ageing, such as loss of balance and eyesight, cause an accident. For many people, it can take a number of falls to realise what has happened to their physical state.

As you get older, many changes can happen gradually so that you tend not to notice them.

Adjusting your routine

Once you become conscious of the physical changes that are occurring in your body, you can adjust your routine to preserve your independent lifestyle. We now know that we can counteract the adverse effects of ageing and inactivity by learning to accommodate helpful activities into our daily life, both around the home and in the community. With safer modifications, you will be better prepared for any tricky situation that could potentially cause a fall.

Home hazards

You can start by making your own environment safer. If you become more aware of fall hazards as you move about each day, and more prepared for avoiding these hazards, you will reduce your risk of falling.

meet Josephine

Josephine got up late one night to go to the toilet, but she had forgotten to leave a light on. She was in a hurry, so instead of fumbling for the switch, she thought she would be okay to just feel her way in the dark. When she got to the bathroom, she turned and sat down quickly, releasing her bladder at the same time. It wasn't until she started to fall that she realised there was no seat under her.

Josephine had misjudged the position of the toilet completely. She threw her hands out to the sides in response but she had already lost her balance. Her head hit the tiled wall and her back slammed against the hard curve of the bathtub. Now in a state of shock, with her limbs sprawled out awkwardly, she desperately groped around in the dark for something to hold on to. Unable to pull herself up, she felt powerless and frightened.

Josephine lay there for what seemed like ages, trying to find something to grasp. Finally, she managed to take off her nightgown and, after many laboured attempts, wrap it around the bathtub taps to gradually pull herself up.

Josephine eventually recovered from the initial shock and the cut to the head, but the event left her with large bruises all over her body and her back seemed to ache more and more each day. Worst of all, she began to fear her own abilities. She'd lost the confidence to carry out her normal daily routines because of the anxious feeling she had about falling.

COMMENT

For Josephine, a variety of factors could have contributed to her fall. Perhaps she had incontinence problems. Maybe it was just because she failed to turn on a light or her balance was not good. Then again, she might not have fallen if she had been able to keep an upright posture, or been strong enough to regain control before she lost her balance.

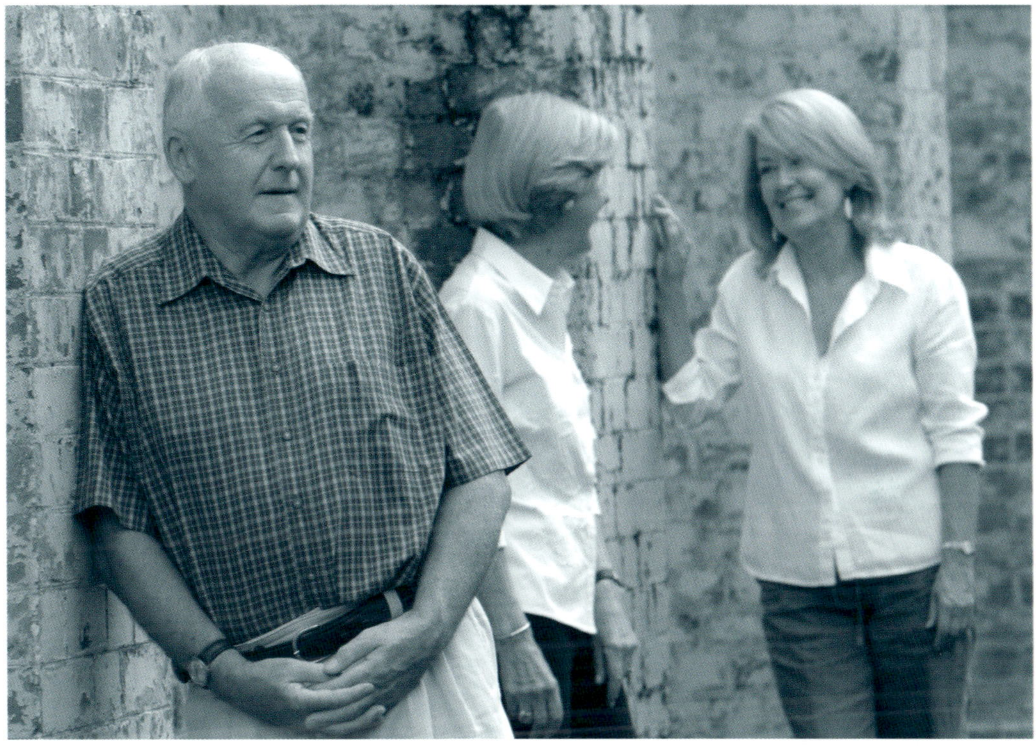

THINK A MOMENT

So what could Josephine have done to better handle this situation? Perhaps she needed:

- a medical check-up to find out about her incontinence
- to avoid drinks after dinner
- a safer lighting system at night with an automatic light source, such as a plug-in night-light. This gives a soft light and you don't have to remember to turn it on
- to ask her doctor for a referral to an eye specialist so she could have her eyes checked for cataracts
- a balance and strength program

These changes would have given Josephine the confidence to feel more in control, which in turn would have reduced her chances of falling.

CHAPTER 3

a quick wrap-up

In Parts 2 and 3, we will take you through some physical, environmental and attitudinal ways to actively reduce your risk of falls. We'll give you practical advice covering the following strategies:

Physical

- improving muscle strength in your legs and hips
- improving your balance
- having regular vision check-ups
- having your medications reviewed, particularly if you take more than one
- cutting down your reliance on tranquillisers and anxiety medications
- trying behavioural alternatives for better sleep
- understanding the importance of vitamin D and calcium in making muscles and bones stronger
- investigating the causes of any postural dizziness as soon as you notice it.

Environmental

- being more aware of fall hazards in and around your home and how to reduce them
- identifying the features of a safe shoe and avoiding footwear that is worn out or dangerous
- recognising poorer vision and how to adjust to it
- moving about safely in the community
- using public transport safely
- learning about hip protectors as an insurance policy against injury.

The journey you are about to embark on will be involving and challenging.

Attitudes and beliefs

- having a realistic awareness of risk
- knowing how to deal with risk
- building up your self-confidence when you do your daily activities
- getting out and about in your community with confidence.

There is one more very important factor to be added to the list: a positive, constructive, realistic attitude towards falls reduction and a belief in your own ability to take control of your life.

A new journey to health

Despite how simple it may seem, making conscious changes to your lifestyle is never easy. The journey you are about to embark on will be involving and challenging. At a basic level, you may question the thoughts and beliefs you hold about yourself and how you live your life. You may evaluate your current choices and compare them to the pros and cons of making changes in order to ensure your future safety and independence. It's about shedding old habits and taking on some new ones.

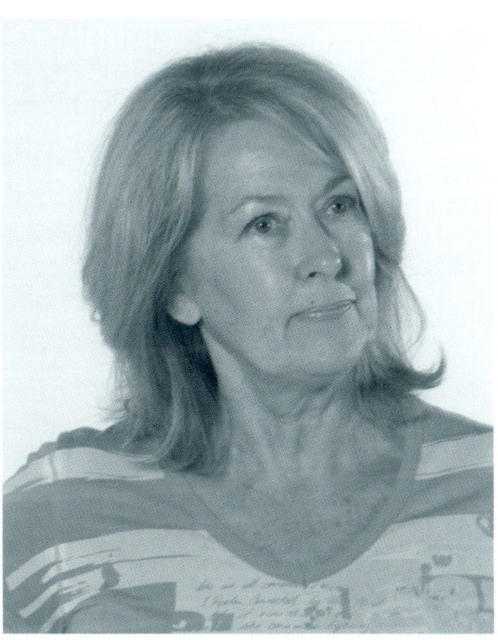

You need to be determined and confident about your own abilities to embark on this journey towards better health

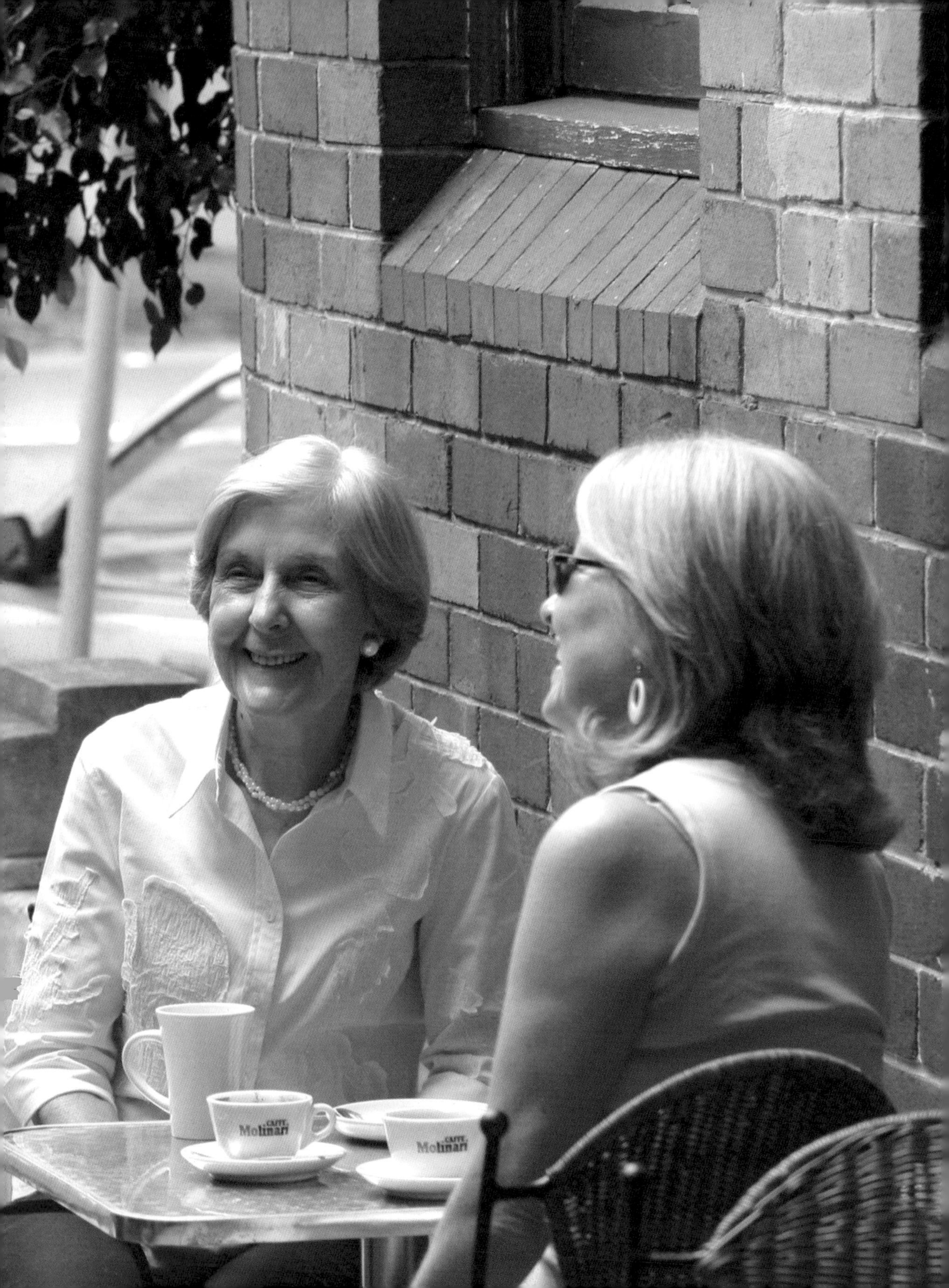
CAFFE Molinari
CAFFE Molinari

PART 2

boosters and barriers to a safer lifestyle

CHAPTER 4

an ongoing process, not just one decision

If a preventive approach to a health problem is shown to work, then using it is just commonsense, especially in the case of falls reduction. It stands to reason that by simply making some changes to your lifestyle, you should be able to lessen the risk of falls.

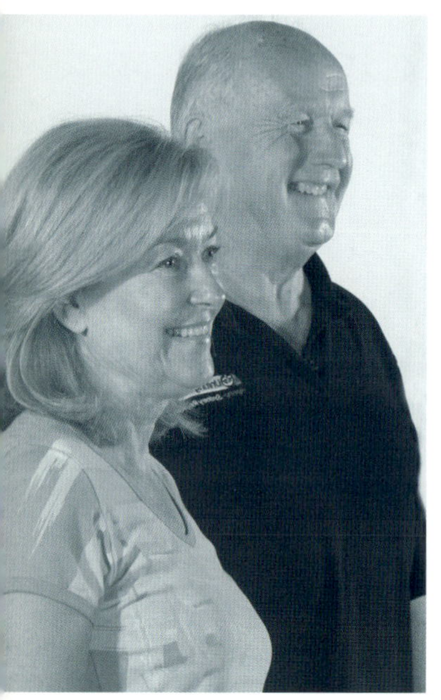

Once you decide to make some positive changes to your life, your whole outlook can change

These simple changes could protect you from the ongoing traumas that can all stem from one accident, as well as the physical and emotional distress and the significant medical costs. While the decision to make some changes might seem easy to make, the truth is that the process of achieving conscious and effective changes to your lifestyle is never so straightforward.

Although falls reduction might not cost a lot in money terms (especially when compared to hospital bills), there is a time cost involved. You will need to invest a reasonable amount of time and energy if your attempts are to have an effect. So falls reduction should not be seen as just one decision, but as an ongoing process where you develop an awareness of risk and a constructive attitude.

It seems just commonsense, but will it really work?

In essence, our research into falls reduction is founded on a collection of practical strategies from many health disciplines including geriatric medicine, physiotherapy and occupational therapy.

Yet despite the research that underpins them, these strategies are pretty uncomplicated. In fact, you already know many of the things you could do to prevent falls.

But if these strategies are so obvious and so effective, why doesn't everyone use them? One reason is that they are not as obvious as we may think. While you might have an intuitive sense of what causes someone to fall, the steps you need to take to address those causes are not always clear. Many older people may not be aware of the various risk factors so it follows that they would see no real need to act.

However, most older people have either had a fall themselves or know people who have. It's therefore much more likely that older people do know about the risks of falling but perhaps choose to ignore these risks, for fear of losing their independence and freedom.

The process of making conscious and effective changes to your lifestyle is never straightforward.

Understanding falls prevention

"Falls prevention" is an unfamiliar term to most people. If you are puzzled by the concept of prevention, you are not alone—it can take a while to fully comprehend what it really means. The ideas in this book will help to make falls prevention clearer for you.

CHAPTER 5

barriers to reducing falls

Now we will look at some of the barriers that could prevent you from reducing your falls risk. We'll help you recognise these barriers and show you some ways to overcome them. You will then be able to get the most out of the practical information in Part 3—to focus not on what you can't do, but on what you can do, and how.

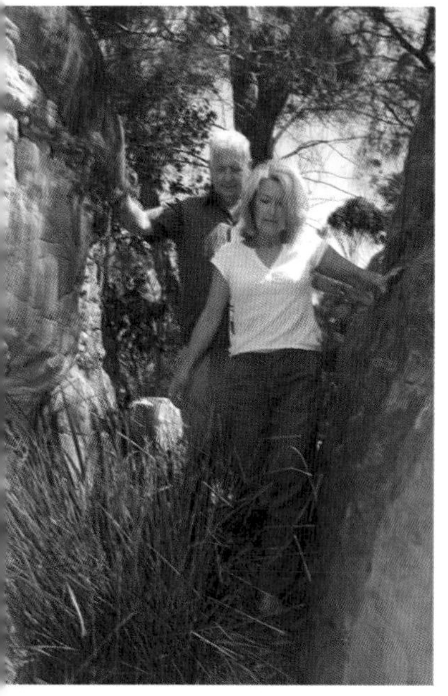

With a healthy attitude, you can explore the great outdoors with confidence

Beliefs about falls

Our society seems to cling to various beliefs about falls, and in particular, beliefs about the relationship between falls and older age. These beliefs can be negative, counterproductive or even just plain false. People involved in the field of falls reduction now have plenty of evidence to prove that these "beliefs" are really just myths. As a society, we still do not fully realise just how steeped in misinformation and prejudice many of these beliefs are. Too many people think the myths about falls and ageing are just commonsense, so they don't question them.

The influence of ageism

Most of these myths are grounded in ageism—a form of discrimination that involves stereotypes, attitudes and thought patterns that discriminate unfairly against the older person.

Some social commentators have written that ageism in western society is a result of the fears that younger people have about growing older and about their own mortality. Unable or unwilling to face these challenges, they promote a culture where older people are sidelined, instead of being afforded the rightful respect that their experience and wisdom in years deserves.

Dispelling the myths

Myths are stories shared by a group. They are part of our personal belief system about the way things are. A number of myths follow that are socially accepted as "truths" yet are really "untruths". As such, they create barriers to us believing that we can create change, and they therefore prevent us from doing something about our situation. So let's challenge some of these myths and misconceptions.

Too many people think the myths about falls and ageing are just commonsense, so they don't question them.

MYTH 1:
Falls are accidents that are beyond our control
The word "fall" is commonly related to the notion of an accident, with the underlying implication that accidents are events beyond our control. When we think of a fall, we think almost automatically that it was "out there", waiting to happen. Most people, when asked what they think causes people to fall, usually blame something external, be it unstable ground, being bumped by another person, the edge of a paver sticking up and so on. Perhaps we tend towards such thinking because it places us beyond the scope of responsibility; if we don't cause the falls, then we can't be blamed.

Although this is a common response, in many ways this kind of thinking is somewhat absurd. Regardless of who or what is to blame, the only person who has to live with the full trauma is the person who has actually fallen. We now know that falls are not just simple, externalised accidents but complex events with a range of contributing factors.

> You can't do much about the larger forces of the world but you can most definitely change the way you approach them.

Of course, there will always be forces beyond our control that may cause us to fall, so this book doesn't claim that falls can be completely avoided. However, research shows that being aware of your risk and learning prevention strategies can make a significant difference. Sure, you can't do much about the larger forces of the world but you can most definitely change the way you approach them. Thinking that you can't do anything about falls because they are caused independently of you is counterproductive and, in fact, false.

MYTH 2:
Having a fall means you are losing your mind

There is a stigma in our society that having a fall in older age proves to friends, family and the world that you are starting to psychologically deteriorate. The belief, rarely spoken about openly, dictates that a person who falls is no longer mentally fit, is unable to look after him or herself and should therefore be shuffled off to professional care so that the accident doesn't happen again.

Having a fall does not mean that you are becoming confused or that you are "losing your mind". A whole range of contributing factors can cause a fall.

MYTH 3:
As you grow older, falls become inevitable

There is an assumption that as we grow older, our body winds down. We become weaker and less stable on our feet, and because these processes of ageing are inevitable, falls must also be inevitable. Statistics show that the chances of having a fall are indeed higher for older people than for the average population. The older you get, the greater your risk

Right: External factors alone, such as an obstacle on a path, don't cause falls. Your mental attitude and physical wellbeing play a large part

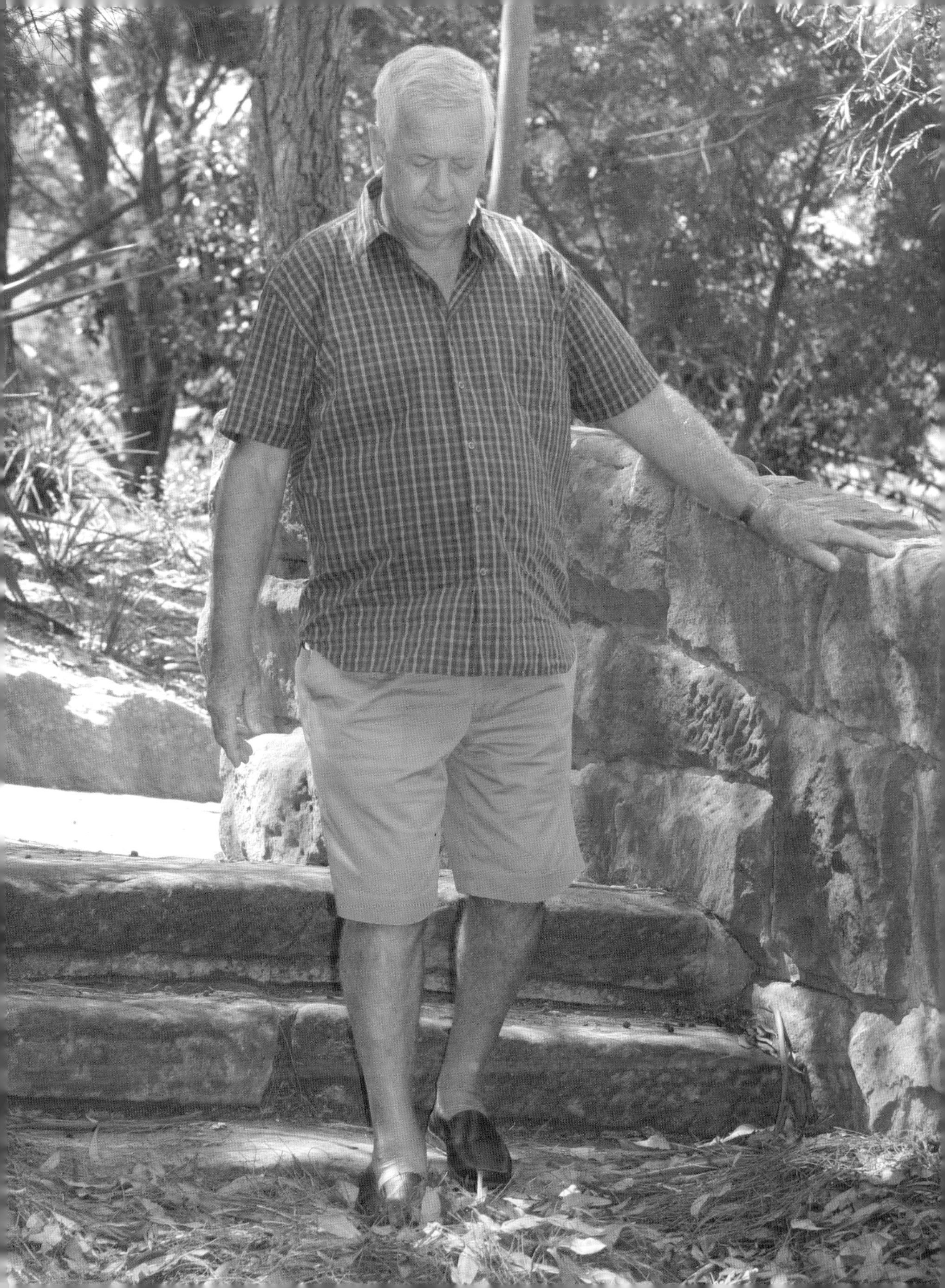

is of falling. It is true that 30 to 40 per cent of people over seventy had a fall last year. But this also means that 60 to 70 per cent in that age group did not fall.

The process of ageing involves physical and psychological changes that can occur quite slowly, without us really noticing. So if we continue to approach our life in the way we always have, the chances of us having a fall will increase as we age. In fact, as we get older, our increasingly inactive lifestyle and how it affects our bodies is one of our major hurdles. The saying "If we don't use it, we lose it" is true. There are many ways to reduce, for example, the physical effects of declining muscle use during the ageing process.

As we get older, our increasingly inactive lifestyle and how it affects our bodies is one of our major hurdles.

MYTH 4:
Older people aren't able to change their ways

Everyone's heard the saying, "You can't teach an old dog new tricks". Such attitudes are almost entirely grounded in stereotypes and misinformation. Older people are often thought of as being stuck in their ways, unable to learn modern methods.

In fact, when developing the Stepping On program, we noticed this kind of stereotyping, even in the attitudes of young health-professional students. People who share this belief tend to underestimate their own abilities and limit their potential. Comments made by older people often reflect a belief that they will have difficulty learning because of their age. This notion only supports negative expectations.

We have found that many older people (just like many younger people) have a great capacity for learning and change. Like all learners, older people just need the opportunity for deeper-level learning, for reflection and for practice and skills development.

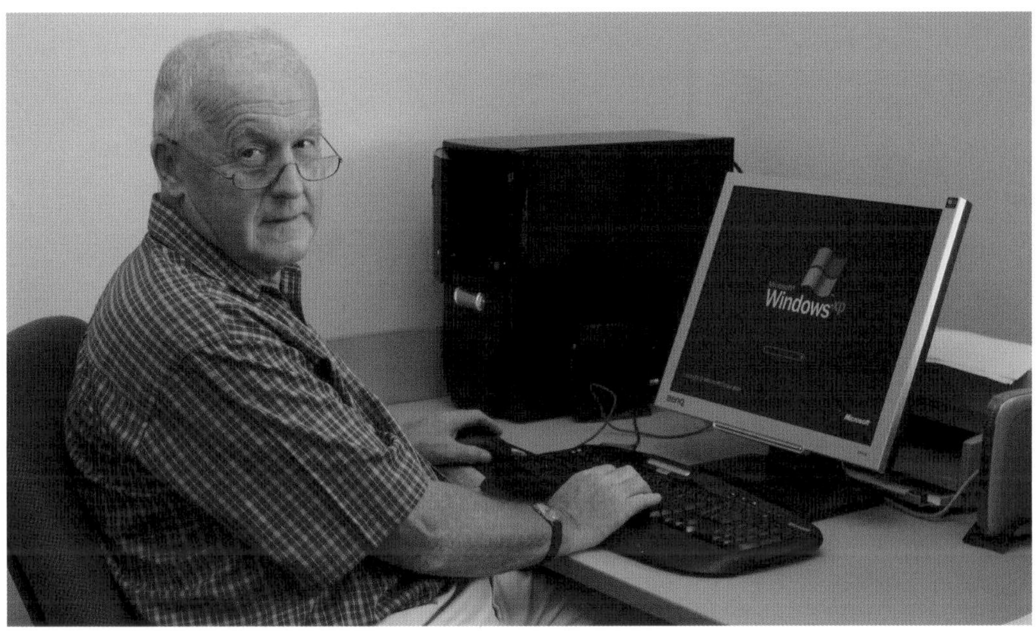

More older people than ever are embracing new technology

> Like all learners, older people need the opportunity for deeper-level learning.

Older people's ability for analytic, creative and practical skills continues to match those of younger adults. But so often, programs designed to teach older people how to approach health issues have not always taken into account the special requirements of the older learner.

Recent studies have shown that much of the difficulty faced by the older person when trying to learn and adapt to new ideas is merely sensory, to do with the senses of sight and hearing. For example, if you have a hearing impairment, a noisy environment will be distracting and will impact on your ability to comprehend and recall more complex material.

There are also suggestions that older people learn best when learning is self-paced, with times for breaks, and that optimism and positive feedback are important. In fact, all these things enhance learning in any age group.

CHAPTER 6

turning decisions to action

The first step to falls prevention is accepting that you can do something about falls, that they are not necessarily a natural part of ageing and that you can learn to make changes.

"Your body deteriorates without you really knowing. It just happens slowly." JAMES

When designing a sound approach to falls prevention, our aim was to draw together workable strategies and present them in practical ways that would also give a feeling of control and self-confidence. The result is a five-step framework from which to start.

The five-step framework

Our approach looks at reducing falls through a framework of questions that create five steps:

1. What are the causes and consequences of falls?
2. What can you do to try to prevent falls?
3. How can you implement these changes?
4. What are the barriers to these changes?
5. How can you overcome the barriers and get positive results?

1. What are the causes and consequences of falls?

A range of environmental, mental and physical factors can cause falls and they can seriously affect our physical and psychological wellbeing. These causes are now well known, and through programs such as Stepping On, the consequences are more likely to be avoided. Yet to reduce your own falls risk, you need to be aware of the risk in your own individual circumstances, so give this some thought.

meet James

James was known in the community for having a busy lifestyle. He was proud of his appearance and loved "keeping up" with younger people. This 75-year-old had had a number of smaller falls in the past, but he was still very confident about his mobility, always rushing about and having no second thoughts about climbing ladders or running down stairs. It wasn't until a Monday morning when the falls became a serious problem. That morning, in his hurry to catch his bus, an uneven piece of the footpath caught James's foot and he tripped. The earth suddenly slipped out from under him and his body plunged headfirst into the gutter. When he fell, he fractured his upper arm, close to the shoulder joint. Bleeding and in a state of shock, he was taken off in an ambulance.

During his time in hospital, James cursed that broken concrete but his thoughts about why the fall happened didn't progress any further than that. It was just an accident, a part of life, so he thought. Then, a few weeks later, he fell again. This time it was a young child suddenly changing direction who made him fall; he saw it as just another accident. And then a few weeks later, another fall. It was only after this third fall that James realised he had to think seriously about what was happening.

COMMENT

James was proud of his independence and it took a while for him to realise that, in order to preserve it, he would have to acknowledge that his body had aged. He noticed that his balance was nowhere near as stable as it had been, and the muscles in his legs were not getting any stronger. Rushing through the uneven urban environment had only heightened these risks. He also realised that he had been shuffling his feet as he walked.

James also knew he had glaucoma, but he wouldn't admit how much he had conditioned himself to ignore it. He suffered from "tunnel vision", meaning he could only see what he was focusing on at any one time. Once he had taken all this in, James wasn't surprised that he had fallen so badly.

Goals for this week

1. Improve light in bedroom
   - [ ] Ring Handyman to trim hedge
   - [ ] Buy light globes ring son to change
2. Do exercises three times a week.
   - [ ] 3 balance exercises
   - [ ] 3 strength exercises

If you share your goals with someone else, you will be more committed to achieving them

2. What can you do to try to prevent falls?

You've thought about what makes falls happen, but what preventive measures are there for falls? What can you do to stop them occurring? Part 3 sets out strategies to reduce your falls risk based on evidence from scientific research. Each of the topics runs through the practical approaches we suggest you could take, depending on your own personal risks and situation.

3. How can you implement these changes?

Now that you've decided what needs to be done, you need a practical framework which will allow you to achieve results. You need to plan, break things down into small, manageable steps, set specific but realistic goals for yourself and create opportunities that will allow you to achieve them through practice.

An integral part of planning is to make a list of the steps you will need to take. First, think about where you are heading and then break down the journey into small, manageable steps. This will prevent you getting overwhelmed by what is ahead and, more importantly, it will make it easier to stay on track.

Break down the journey into small, manageable steps.

SETTING GOALS

In the world of business, education and health, much has been written about the benefit of specific planning to get better results. Part of this process is goal setting. Goals are essential for making changes in our lives, and the goals you set need to be quite specific. Your overall objective might be to stop falls, but the goals to achieve this must be tangible, doable and stated in very certain terms. If a goal is expressed too vaguely, it will be lost.

meet Barbara

Barbara had a big fall in the supermarket. Walking along the aisle and looking at the products on the shelves, she failed to see a grape that was lying on the floor in front of her. Unfortunately, she stepped right on top of it. Her foot slipped out from under her and she landed on her back. She had to be wheeled out of the supermarket on a stretcher.

During her long stay in hospital, Barbara received a spinal fusion operation. This left her back much weaker than it had been, and she was in considerable pain throughout the recovery. When she got out of hospital she couldn't drive the car and wasn't even confident enough to go to the shops by herself. This was a big problem for Barbara. Her husband had just entered a nursing home and she now needed to cope with living alone in a new flat. What's more, she was in an unfamiliar community where she didn't know many people and she wasn't used to the local environment.

COMMENT

In order to manage by herself and prevent any more falls, Barbara needed to address the risks that were stopping her from living confidently. Her husband moving away had left her feeling downhearted, and she felt isolated in her new community where people came from very different backgrounds to her.

It was very unlucky for Barbara that the grape was on the ground, but it was largely her own responsibility to look out for her own safety. She just hadn't been concentrating on where she was walking.

After the incident, Barbara remembered a number of recent times around her new home, such as going down the stairs and reaching for things in high kitchen cupboards, when she hadn't felt as confident as she used to. She recognised she wasn't as sure on her feet in public either, often standing still in large crowds to let people move around her instead of choosing her own safe path.

Perhaps Barbara's sense of uncertainty and lack of confidence had added to her distraction and compounded her risk of falling. Barbara needs to set goals to make changes in her life.

"All of these changes in my life had made me a bit unsettled. I felt as though my life was becoming out of my own control, and it used to worry me greatly. The fall only made this feeling worse."

BARBARA

Some goals look too far into the future—you need to know when a goal will be accomplished to know exactly what you are aiming for. "Walking more often" is unclear and has no time limit on it, but "walking to the shops before lunch three times a week" is specific and measurable. By stating exactly what you will do and by setting a time period, you will know whether you have achieved it or not.

Each goal must also be relevant. You need to make the goals personally realistic in order to achieve the outcomes you want, and you need to feel that if you reach them, you will change your habits. Your goals must be reasonable and phrased as very specific behaviours or actions that relate to particular situations. For example, "being more physically active" is not a behaviour but "climbing the steps instead of using the escalator" is; "having less clutter in my bedroom" is not an action but "putting my shoes in the wardrobe straightaway" is.

To help reach a certain goal, think about it in terms of an action plan. By breaking down the goal into manageable steps, you may turn commitment into action as Maggie does on page 37.

4. What are the barriers to implementing these changes?

You now know in more practical terms what can be done to reduce your falls risk. And yet, it is likely that there will still be barriers to your success. No-one has complete control over their behaviour, especially when a routine is involved. That is why we encourage you to think about your own barriers before you get to them, so you are more prepared and ready to overcome them.

When you decide to adapt your lifestyle, you make many decisions. It helps to weigh up the advantages and disadvantages of your proposed action by writing down the "pros" and "cons" in a clear way. The best way to do this is on a "balance sheet", where you list the pros and cons in two columns. This will make you more aware of the positive outcomes, and will also highlight some of the barriers you might encounter. If you can recognise the barriers when you are faced with them, you will be better prepared to overcome them.

Planning in small steps makes it easier to stay on track.

5. How can you overcome the barriers so that you get results?

Even though you might set out with the utmost optimism and enthusiasm, things don't always go as planned. It is quite common to have a "relapse". This is where you slip back into old ways, be it due to old habits, forgetting your plan, not having the energy, not yet feeling convinced you need to do all this, and so on.

Re-evaluating your goals and restating your action plans

As you improve and as you encounter new barriers, you need to keep evaluating your goals and updating your action plans. You are not making New Year's resolutions here. It is an ongoing process that continues over time.

We found that a period of seven to eight weeks is essential for getting the strategies properly in place. This time frame will be about right for getting your personal routine in place, too. After about three months, it's good to review and reflect on the obstacles you have overcome and on your achievements and progress. Identify your personal risks and decide what you need to do to keep reducing them. Also identify your barriers so you

meet Maggie

Maggie has been doing her balance and strength exercises (see Part 3) and is feeling more confident now to cope with walking around her local area. She has decided to increase her physical activity by walking more often. She has also become aware that many of the busiest parts of her home are dimly lit.

COMMENT

Maggie needs to set a goal for each of her realisations by formulating answers to the three questions below:

- What exactly will Maggie do?
- When will Maggie do it?
- How often will Maggie do it?

This table shows the goals Maggie has set:

ACTION	• walk more often • improve the lighting in the dimly lit parts of the house
WHAT EXACTLY WILL MAGGIE DO?	• walk to the shops • use higher-wattage globes in her lounge and hall. Put it on the shopping list now
WHEN WILL MAGGIE DO IT?	• before lunch • get the globes on the next shopping trip and ask her neighbour to change them when he visits her next time
HOW OFTEN WILL MAGGIE DO IT?	• three times this week • keep a spare bulb so it's ready when needed

So Maggie's walking goal becomes "to walk to the shops before lunch three times this week". Once Maggie defines her goal in specific terms, she can monitor her accomplishments. When she communicates clearly with herself, she is able to re-evaluate her goals and reward herself when she accomplishes them—even if the reward is just praise.

meet Gracie

A major goal for Gracie was to have a regular vision check-up. So she made a balance sheet listing the pros and cons of making an appointment with the optometrist every year. This was her list:

PROS

- I'll know that my eyes are disease-free
- My glasses will be the most suitable strength for my eye condition
- I will feel in control of my health
- I'm making sure my vision doesn't degenerate without me knowing about it
- I'll have a sense of security about my vision
- I'll be able to move about with safety, especially outdoors
- I'll be able to keep up my reading, needlework etc
- It will be easier to do my banking and read business cards
- I know I am looking after myself and can then keep caring for my husband.

CONS

- It takes time
- I'm too busy to organise it
- It costs money
- It will probably interfere with my social life
- How would I get there?
- The eye drops make it hard for me to see afterwards
- It's too hard to get someone to help me after using the eye drops
- I don't want to ask the family for help
- I look after my husband and can't get away
- I babysit the grandchildren and don't have time.

"Eventually, I had to ask myself: what is more important? My safety and comfort, or fancy shoes?"
AUDREY

recognise them and are ready to overcome them. Establish the pros and cons of your new decisions and develop an action plan to assess how you are tracking.

Simple cues to jog your memory

No matter how good your intentions, sometimes you just forget to follow through, especially if you're trying to fit new adjustments into your normal routine. So use reminders to help you remember:

- place notes on the fridge, by the phone, on the mirror or next to your chair. These notes can remind you which day is your exercise day, to ask the pharmacist about your new medication, or to make a list of your medications and have it ready in your wallet the next time you visit your doctor. If you have something special to do when next you go out, place a reminder note somewhere you will see it as you leave, such as in the hall or on the inside of your front door.

- have your exercise chart on display. Then it's harder to forget about it or ignore it. Some people put their chart or their weights in their living

meet Audrey Audrey had a collection of fancy shoes that she loved, and she made sure she didn't give them away in her de-cluttering campaign. Unfortunately, she was finding that with her sore back, the shoes were no longer practical or safe. She had to walk awkwardly in them to stop her back from hurting, and heel–toe exercises hurt even more. After re-evaluating the situation, she went shopping for some sensible shoes that were safer for her to walk in. They didn't look too bad either!

meet Dawn

Dawn's new unit was much smaller than her old home. She had brought all her belongings with her but now there wasn't enough room for them all, making the house cluttered with half-opened boxes and things everywhere. Apart from looking messy, Dawn realised it wasn't safe to have her unit so full and untidy.

Although it was difficult to part with her possessions, Dawn spent a few days deciding what she could live without and who could take the excess. Then she rang those people and asked them to pick up the things they'd agreed to take, and asked her daughter to help her take anything left over to the tip.

COMMENT

Unlike her old house, the slightly rundown government housing unit she was now living in was not completely suitable. For example, in her new unit, many of the cupboards were too high for her to reach with confidence. Dawn decided to buy a stepladder so she could reach everything without overstretching or wobbling on a chair. She asked her daughter to help her choose a safe, sturdy one from a hardware store and transport it home. Realising that she would be using it regularly, Dawn made an accessible space for it to live beside her fridge in the kitchen.

Another problem with the unit was the poor lighting, especially in the stairway, where the steps were difficult to see. As it was the local council's responsibility to make the block of units safe, Dawn asked them to install brighter fluorescent lights.

And the courtyard, after years of neglect, was now covered in slippery moss. Dawn couldn't get rid of the moss by herself so she asked the council if they could clean that up, too. They eventually came around and did these jobs. Dawn also decided to sweep the courtyard on the first Saturday of every month, to make sure the moss didn't return.

room so they know they'll feel guilty and won't be able to relax properly until they've done the exercises.

Time to make changes

At first you might find your new plans feel a bit awkward in your normal routine. Try linking them with other well-established habits. This is where an action plan is useful. If you can plan to integrate your new decisions into an established routine, you'll find it much easier to remember, to follow through on, and to become accustomed to. For example, think about your best time to do the exercises—while watching TV? When you get up? To change your routine and establish new habits, you usually need to bring the habits into your consciousness for a while until they become entrenched. Keep in mind that this is not easy and it takes time to overcome the setbacks. A seven-week schedule should give you time to adjust to your new routine, so give yourself a reasonable amount of time to get used to your changes and plans.

Give yourself a reasonable amount of time to get used to your changes and plans.

Self-confidence

Confidence in your own abilities is a powerful force. It not only influences what you think you can do, but what you actually can do. We are continually making judgements about our capabilities. It's important to listen to these judgements so that you have a good idea about what you're capable of. However, it's also important to challenge them. Repeated failures can lead to you putting yourself down unnecessarily, which undermines your self-confidence and throws your motivation off course.

But if you continue to struggle and overcome these failures, this will actually boost your self-confidence. If you are unsure of your abilities, build up your confidence by doing things in small, manageable steps.

Positive thinking

Try to be conscious of how you are thinking. This may seem unusual at first. If you are telling yourself that you have failed, review the experience as something to learn from. What can you take from your experience? What could you now do differently? Try to rephrase negative thoughts into positive but realistic statements. You might think this is silly but it does work; encouragement and genuine optimism are infectious. If you fill your mind with positive thoughts in spite of the challenges you face, you are far more likely to overcome them.

If you fill your mind with positive thoughts in spite of the challenges you face, you are far more likely to overcome them.

Give yourself feedback

Review and reflect on what you've done lately—both the good and not-so-good experiences—and how you've gone with them. Make charts of your goals, broken down into smaller practical steps. Give yourself a tick when you've successfully taken a step on the chart. This will help you to get into a routine and give you a sense of achievement, which is important when you are starting something new. Stop and reflect on all your accomplishments, and explore and evaluate your experiences. This will lead to new perspectives and new ways of behaving. Give praise and don't forget to reward yourself when you achieve your goals. Buy some flowers or go to the movies when you have committed to a course of action and you feel like it's underway.

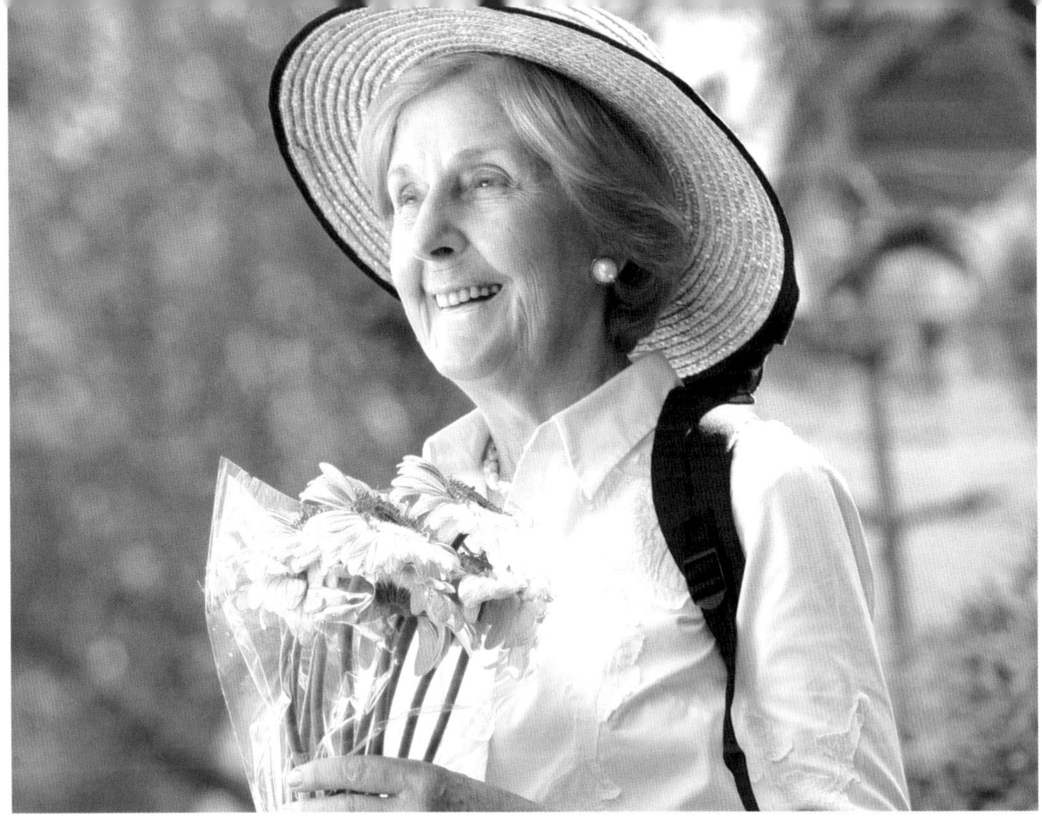

Reward yourself when you feel that a course of action for a healthier lifestyle is underway

Reviewing the five-step framework

Consider these five questions when you are working out your plan to reduce falls:

1. What are the causes and consequences of falls?
2. What can you do to try to prevent falls?
3. How can you implement these changes?
4. What are the barriers to implementing these changes?
5. How can you overcome the barriers and get positive results?

Keep these questions and your answers in mind as you read through Part 3 and use them as an aid to your decision-making process. When considering your own falls-related experiences and the stories you hear, ask yourself these questions to help evaluate the pros and cons for your goals and to get the most out of different safety strategies.

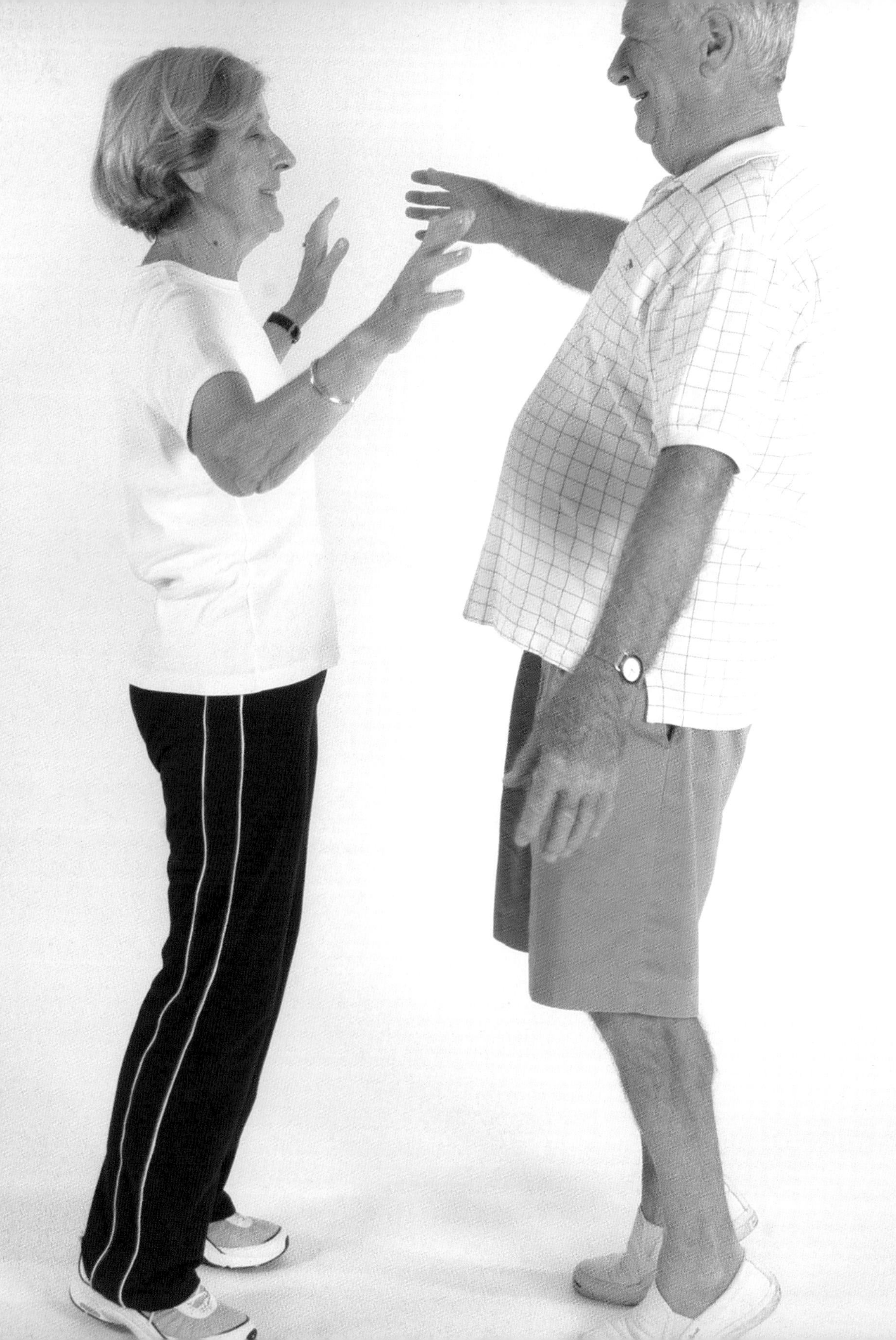

PART 3

how to keep you on your feet

In this part we get down to the detail and give you practical ideas for reducing your risk of falls.

MOVING gives you a set of simple balance and muscle-strengthening exercises, and explains why and how they can help protect you from falling. This set of chapters also introduces ways of moving about safely, such as getting up from a chair, heel–toe walking and climbing stairs.

FEELING SAFE AT HOME AND IN YOUR COMMUNITY helps you become more aware of the fall hazards at home and in your local community. This set of chapters suggests ways to adapt to your environment so you either reduce the hazards or approach them differently.

HOW TO HANDLE A CHANGING BODY covers a range of body issues that influence your falls risk—including changing vision, multiple medications and dizziness—and gives some practical strategies for dealing with these.

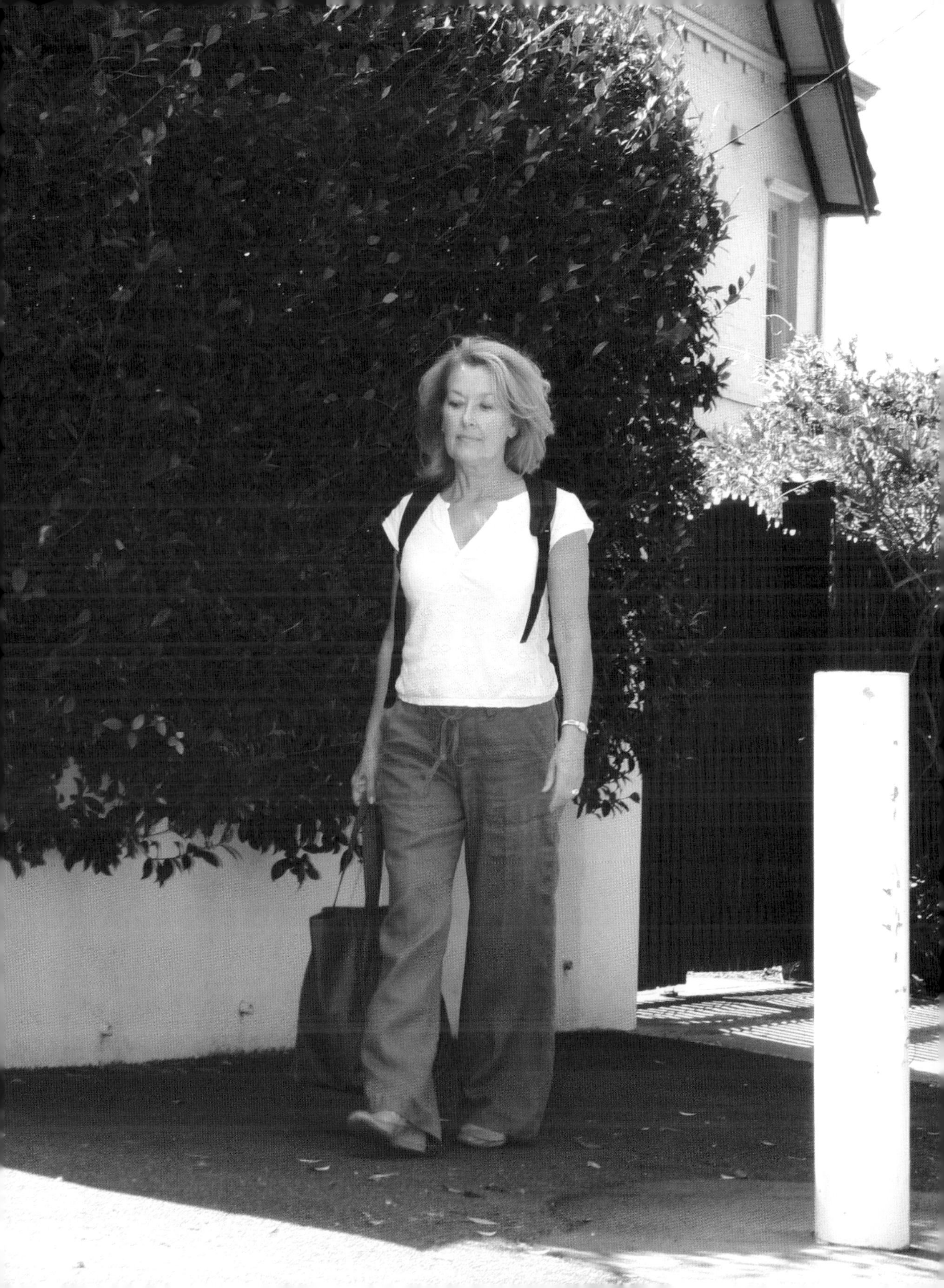

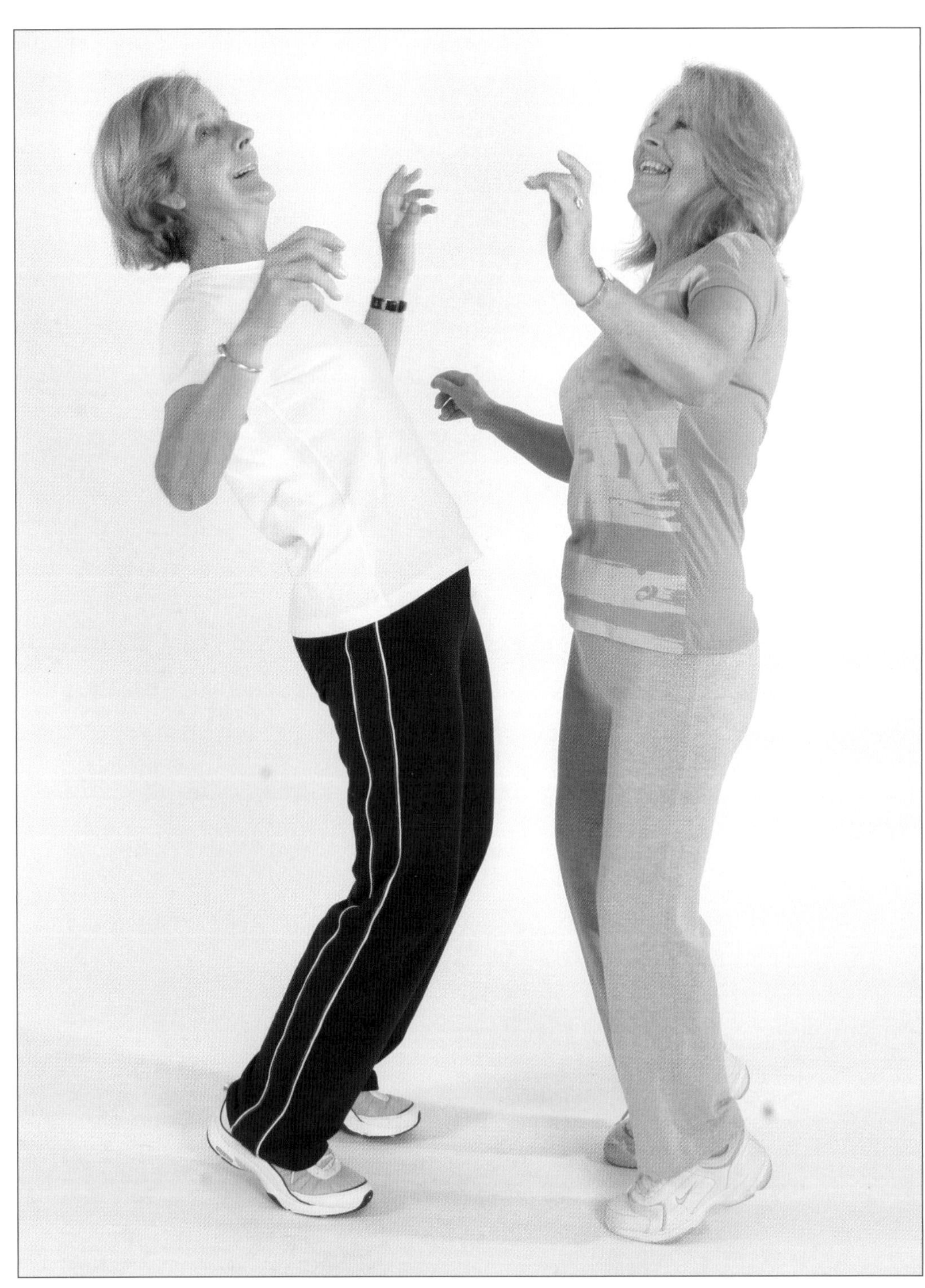

moving

CHAPTER 7

moving about safely

Being able to move about safely is the key to maintaining your independence and doing what you want in your life. The exercises that follow are the basic building blocks to achieve this. They improve your balance and strength, which will reduce your risk of falling.

Once you start to improve your balance and strength, you can then concentrate more on how you actually move around in your environment, both indoors and outdoors. With better balance and strength, you will be able to move around more safely and will be better protected from the risk of falling.

Let's now look at some suggestions to increase our safety while doing basic activities that we all experience frequently.

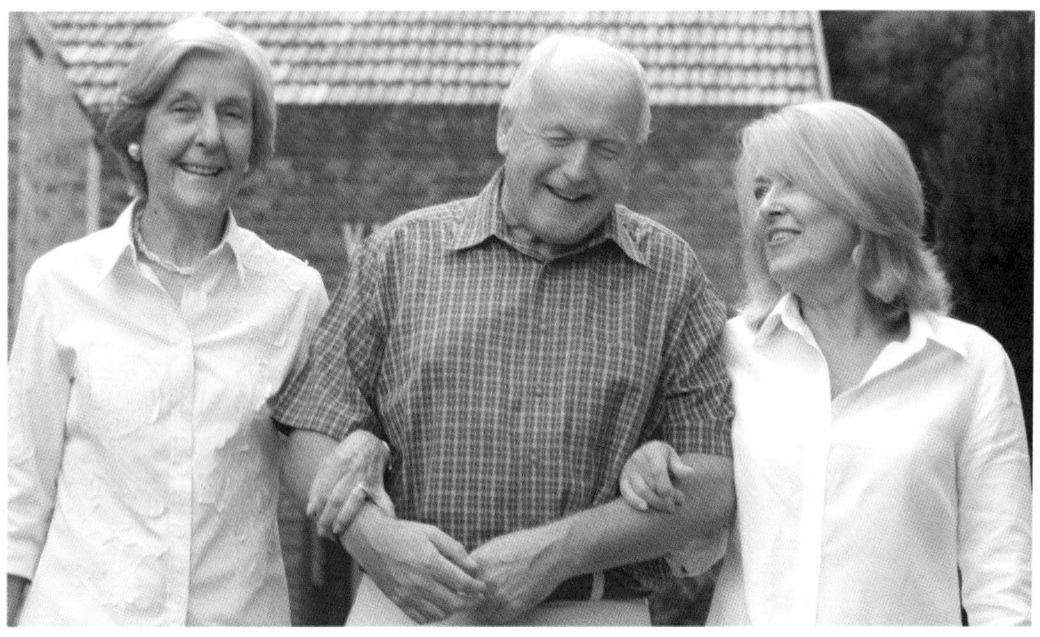

getting up from a chair

- Move your bottom forward in the chair, keeping your feet together and close to the chair legs
- Make sure your knees are in line with your shoulders and are the same distance apart
- Bring your head forward and remember "nose over toes"
- Keeping your head up, push up with both arms if necessary, pausing once you are standing to regain your balance before moving

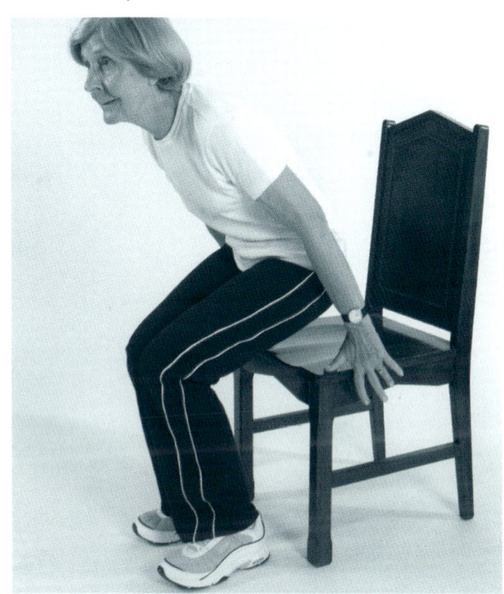

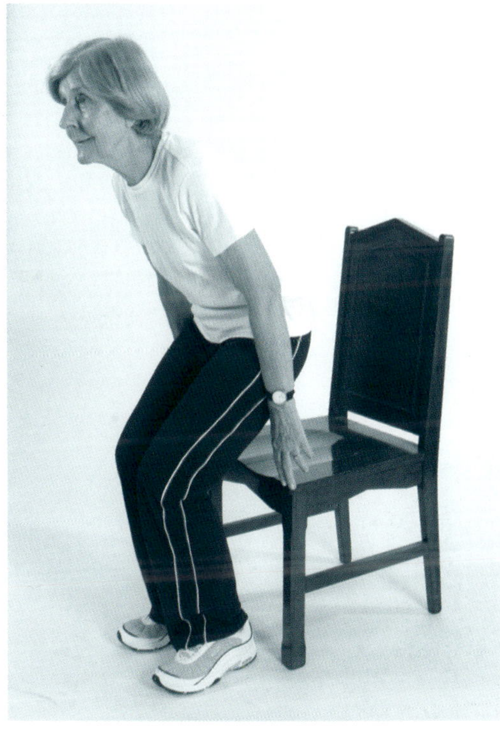

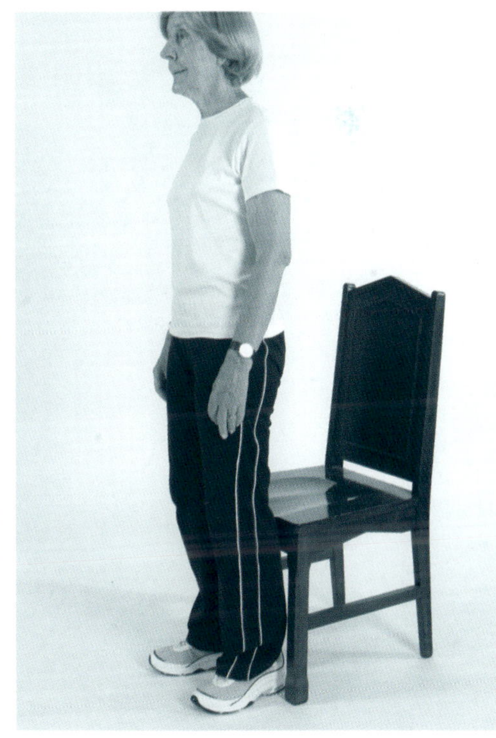

using a walking stick safely

- Adjust your stick for your height. The handle should be level with your wrist when your arm is at your side
- Use your stick in the opposite hand to your affected or weaker leg. When you walk, bring the stick forward at the same time as your weaker leg
- The rubber stopper on the bottom should always be in good condition Renew the stopper when it is worn so that it doesn't slip out from under you

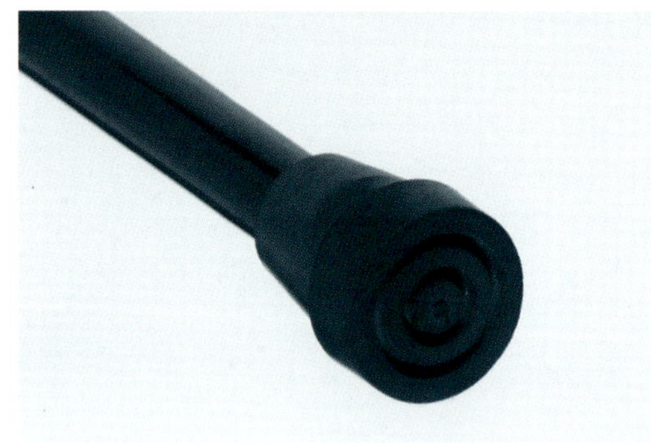

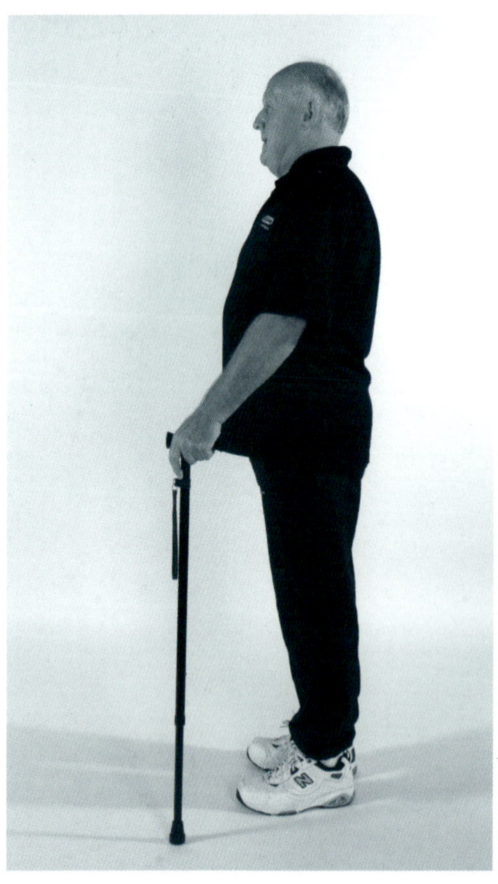

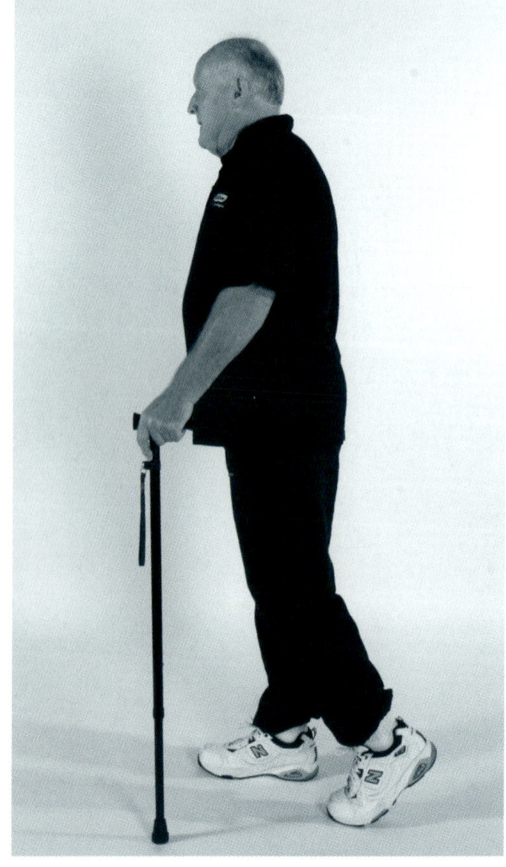

walking on uneven or unfamiliar ground

- Keep your legs a little wider apart to increase your base of support, which will make your centre of gravity lower and more stable
- This is especially useful for ramps and slopes, which can pose quite a challenge for some people

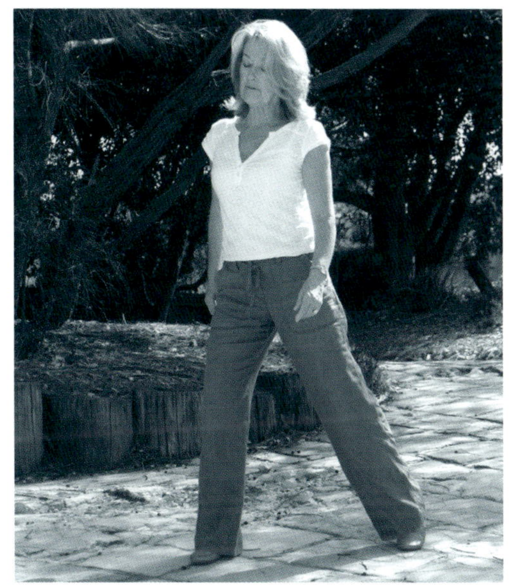

meet Nancy

Nancy has had one fall since she began implementing our recommendations. She was tired and she had tripped over a bag left on the ground. Nancy talked about what she had got out of being in the group. Before the program, she had had quite a few falls outside. She didn't like to walk much, and walked very tensely with her shoulders down and her body stooped over.

Since attending the group, Nancy has found that she scans ahead and does the "heel–toe" walk when she's out and about. She is less tense and less stooped. Neighbours have commented that she has her bounce back in her step. She now enjoys walking again.

COMMENT

Nancy's story is a good example of breaking the cycle. She worked hard to get fitter and as a result, is feeling confident and in control again.

using steps and gutters

- Hold on to a railing for safety if available
- Otherwise, hold on to other props, such as signposts, to help negotiate gutters. Look out for useful street furniture that you may be able to use for support
- If you have one leg stronger than the other, step up first with your stronger leg, and step down first with your weaker leg
- Use a wider base when you are negotiating slopes, kerb ramps and uneven ground. This makes you more stable

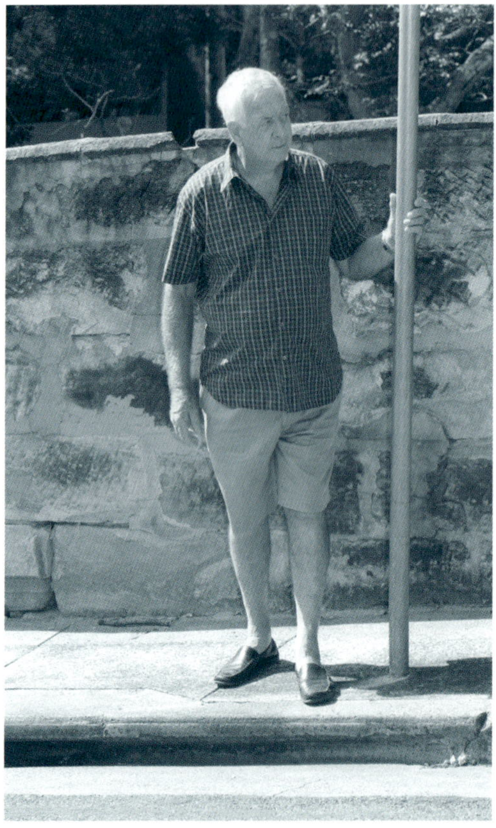

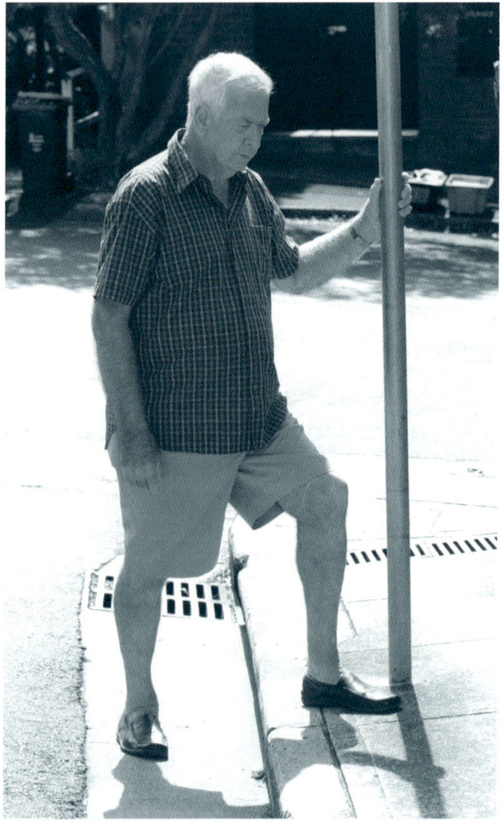

scanning ahead

- Look ahead up to a car length or so (or as far as you are able to see). This helps you to see hazards coming up that may cause you problems, such as cracks and debris on the ground, but still allows you to appreciate your surroundings

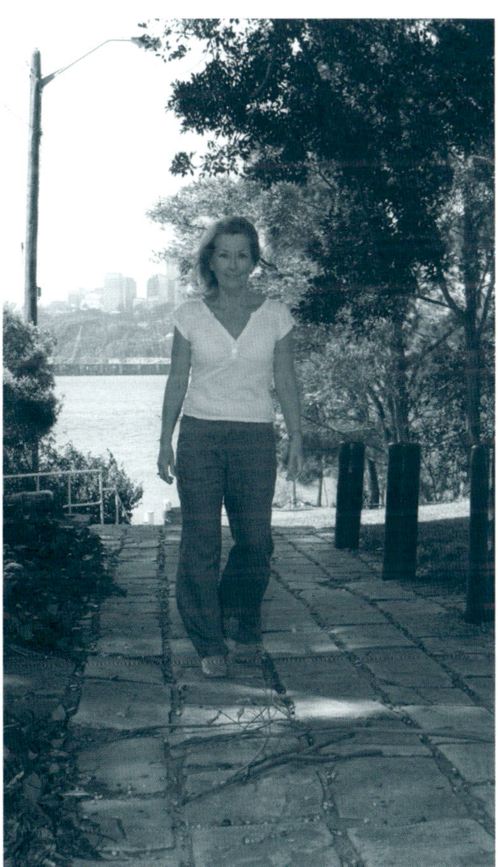

- When you get to the hazard, slow down and look down at it with your eyes while you negotiate it, but keep your head up. As you step off, look straight ahead and start scanning again

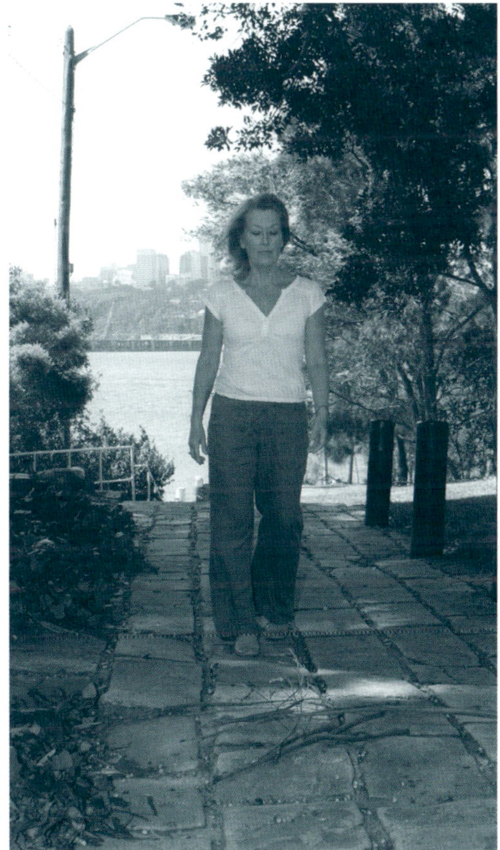

heel–toe walking

- When you take a step, let your heel touch the ground first, smoothly followed by your toe
- Keep your head up, which will help you to scan ahead more easily, too
- Many people look straight down as they walk. Our participants told us that learning to hold their head up and look ahead gave them a great boost of confidence

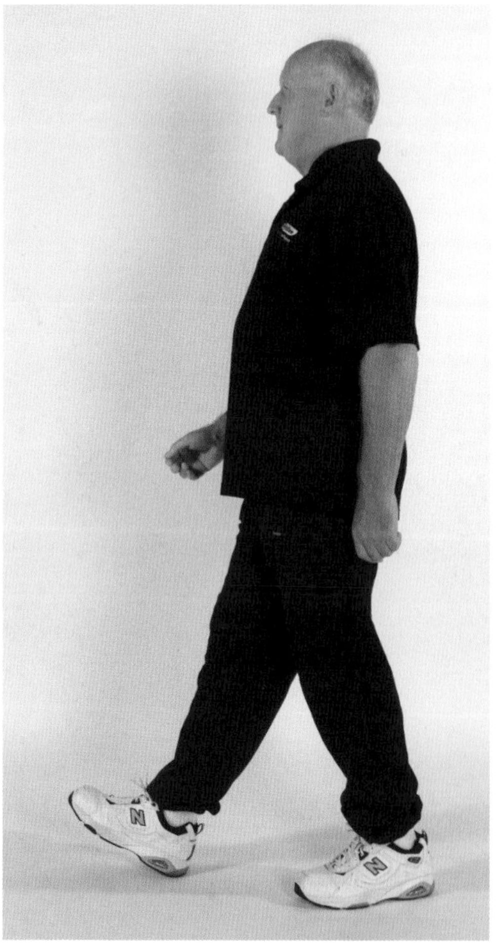

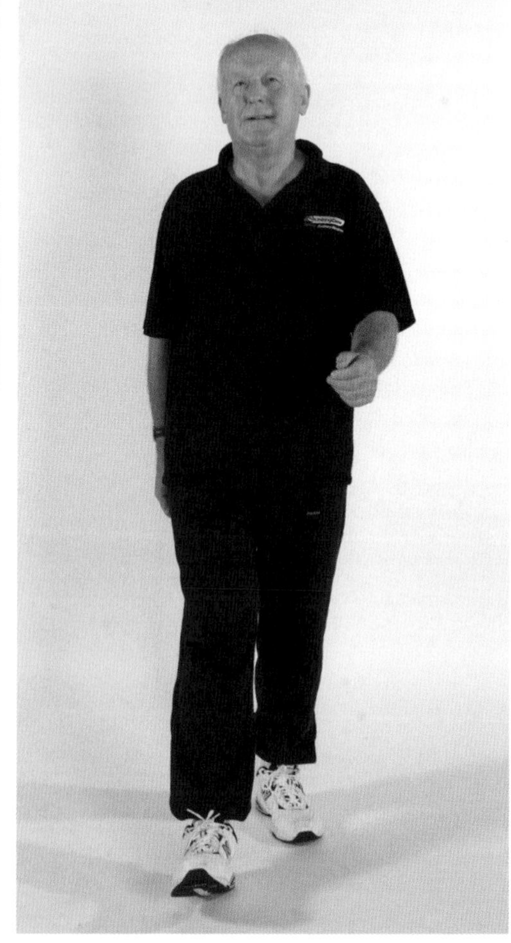

Learning to hold your head up and scan ahead when you walk can give you a great boost of confidence.

Heel–toe walking and scanning ahead

If you walk in a heel–toe sequence rather than shuffling your feet, and you scan ahead, you will have more time to prepare for hazards and changes in ground level. Heel–toe walking and scanning ahead are two of the most helpful tips for preventing falls.

meet Keith

Keith equated walking on uneven ground with driving a vehicle in a hail storm. When you drive in a hail storm, you should be confident that your tyres have a good tread and you look ahead because you never know how far the hail extends. You tend to drive more slowly and you try to steer your wheels along a more stable track in the road. Keith equated always checking the tyre tread with making sure that you have non-slippery soles on your shoes when you walk. And like driving, when you walk on uneven ground, you scan ahead for hazards, you take care to walk with a stable base over rough ground and you choose the safest path.

TRY THIS

Practise heel–toe walking and scanning ahead for just a few minutes each day on level ground. Find ways to challenge yourself. Walk on different floor surfaces and at different gradients, for example, and work up to grassy surfaces, which have a more challenging surface. As your balance and strength improve you will find walking and moving about easier.

CHAPTER 8

balance and strength—an essential combination

There is very strong evidence to show that better balance reduces falls. But to improve your balance and maintain the gains, you need regular practice. The saying "if you don't use it, you lose it" applies to balance, just as it does to muscle strength.

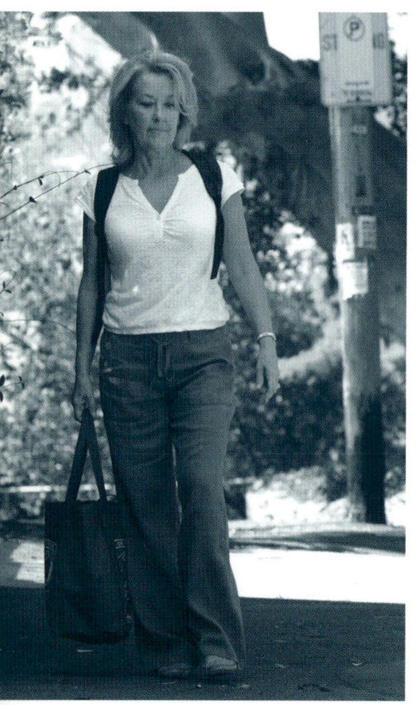

Balance and muscle training are the building blocks for walking confidently and safely

To walk better and be more active, and to do it safely, you need to maintain the muscle strength in your legs as well as your ability to balance. You need to be strong enough to negotiate obstacles and to recover your stability if you lose it momentarily, and have enough confidence in your balance to cope with uneven steps and gutters.

Aerobic fitness benefits your cardiovascular health and, therefore, your capacity for doing daily activities without getting exhausted. However, the most dramatic benefits for maintaining mobility and bodily function are achieved with strength and balance training. It is now accepted that just walking is not sufficient to prevent falls; you also need to load your muscles three times a week by doing activities that offer some resistance to them, and to challenge your balance. Once you are stronger and your balance is better, you will be walking more safely, for longer, and be able to enjoy more physical activity.

A sequence for success

The balance and strength-training exercises in the following chapters are part of an exercise sequence that has been proven to improve balance and strength and to reduce falls. If you do the exercises on a regular basis, you will be able to walk with a strong heel–toe stride and reduce your risk of falling when you go about your everyday activities. If you find any of the exercises too easy or too difficult, or if you experience dizziness or persistent pain, we recommend you see a physiotherapist or health professional who will assist you with a more tailored program.

meet Lorna

Lorna has led a very active life. She has seven children whom she meets up with often, and she loves going to the theatre. Lorna had trouble a couple of times trying to stand up out of the theatre seats, but she was so embarrassed that she didn't tell anyone and just tried to forget about it. Then a few days later, she went to town. It was very rainy and windy. Without warning, Lorna fell flat on her face, badly bruising her eye and jaw. She felt so shattered and jittery from the fall that she went straight to the doctor. She explained to her GP that while she knows that walking is very good for her heart and mental wellbeing, she feels that if she went walking now, she would fall. Lorna feels like she's in a twilight zone and feels panicky. She knows she has to walk to stay healthy and independent but doesn't feel confident doing so because she doesn't know why she fell in the first place. Lorna just doesn't know what to do.

COMMENT

Lorna would really benefit from doing some balance and muscle training. These are the building blocks for walking confidently and safely to prevent falls. It just makes so much sense—if you increase your balance and have stronger ankle, knee and hip muscles, you can then walk more easily and better. Walking is good, but strength and balance training are a great investment for making walking safer.

CHAPTER 9

balance

Balance is the ability to stay upright while standing still, moving about or doing everyday tasks. It also gives you the ability to "catch" yourself when you are about to fall.

When you sense an obstacle is near, you respond by adjusting your posture to avoid it. Our sense of balance is actually very complex. It involves many different muscle groups and is controlled by a particular part of the brain called the cerebellum. Balance is directly related to the integration of two specific brain functions—motor and sensory. Surprising as it may be, you are able to improve your balance through practising some simple exercise routines.

Our sense of balance is actually very complex.

A balancing act

Like all abilities controlled by your brain, improving and maintaining balance requires repetition and constant testing. This allows the pathways in your brain to fire up again and start to rewire themselves, making the connections that will give you back your sense of balance. When you were young, you tested your balance all the time—on bikes and scooters, playing games, walking on fences. It has taken many years for your balance to weaken but some simple daily exercises can fix this.

The motor and sensory pathways that form the basis of your balance can be enhanced through practice. But to do this, the balance tasks need to closely mimic everyday situations. The closer they are to real-life functions, the more likely it is that your improved balance will carry over to situations where you might be at risk of losing your balance and slipping or tripping.

How can we improve balance?

Testing involves pushing your body to the safe limits of what it can achieve, so that it can improve.

To improve balance you have to test your balance. The idea of testing involves pushing your body to the safe limits of what it can achieve, so that it can improve. This also means that over time, as your confidence and skill improve, you will need to slowly progress to more challenging balance activities to continue making gains.

There are many exercises you can use to test and improve your balance, but we have chosen five of the most effective ones to show you. They are easy to do and remember. However, to get an effect, you must keep progressing and upgrading each exercise so that you constantly test your balance. There are also ideas for how you can go about devising your own additional routines.

The five balance exercises are:
- heel–toe (tandem) standing
- heel–toe walking
- finding your toppling point
- heel walking
- sideways walking

Regardless of any other exercise or activity, you should do these five exercises at least three times a week. If you can do them more often, you'll get greater benefit.

THE BALANCE ROUTINE

To improve balance, you need to test your balance. So start at a place with these exercises where you feel you are challenged, but safe. As soon as the exercise is not testing your balance, upgrade to the next level. It's important that you keep progressing.

heel–toe (tandem) standing

In this exercise you keep moving onto your front foot and then your back foot, shifting your weight as you go.

- Stand up tall beside a bench, rail or similar support. Hold on to the support and look ahead
- Place one foot directly in front of the other foot so that your feet form a straight line. (This pose is called the "tandem" position)
- Hold this position for 10 seconds

AN EASIER START

- If you find it hard to balance at first, keep your feet a little further apart

UPGRADE

- Shift your weight alternately from one foot to another
- Change position by moving your back foot from behind to now be in front. Repeat holding the heel–toe position and shifting your weight

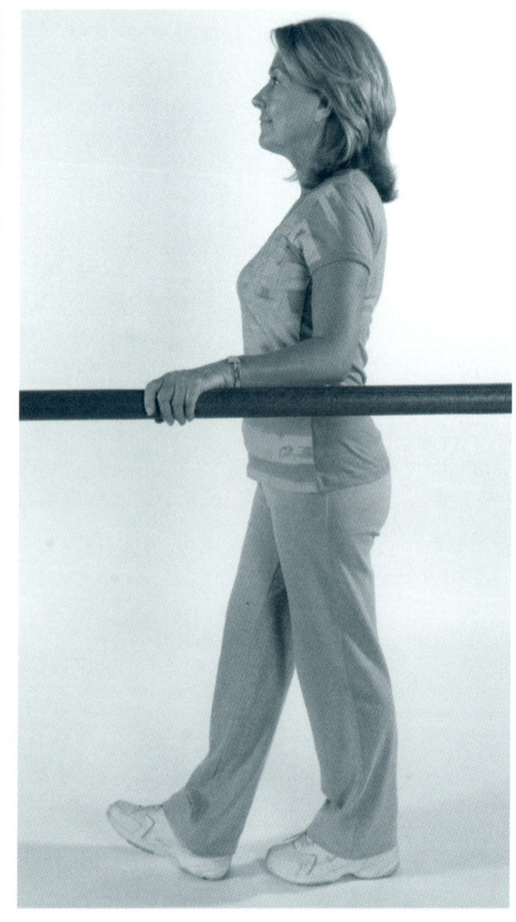

To challenge your balance, shift your weight from one foot to the other

AS YOU PROGRESS

- Hold the heel–toe position, shifting your weight as you do, for longer than 10 seconds
- Hold onto the support with one finger
- Don't hold on
- Try with your eyes closed

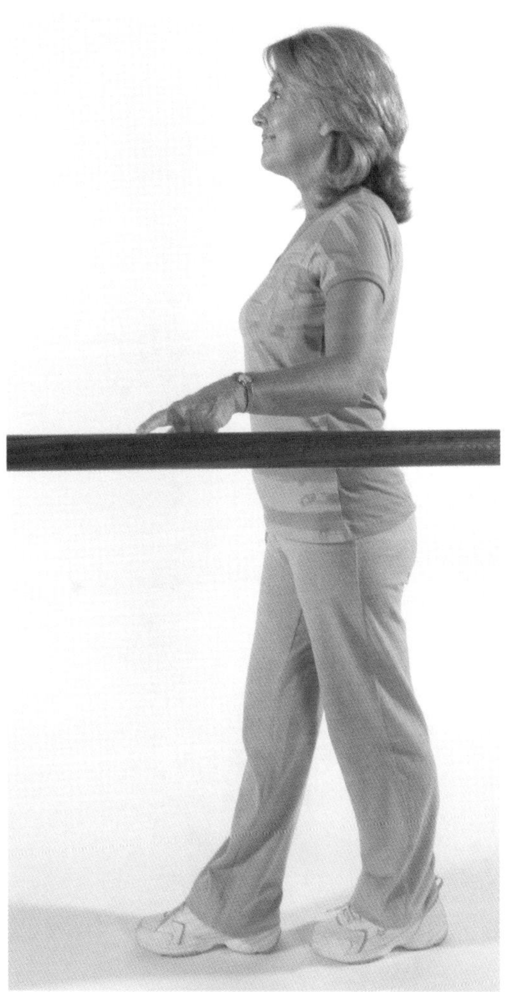

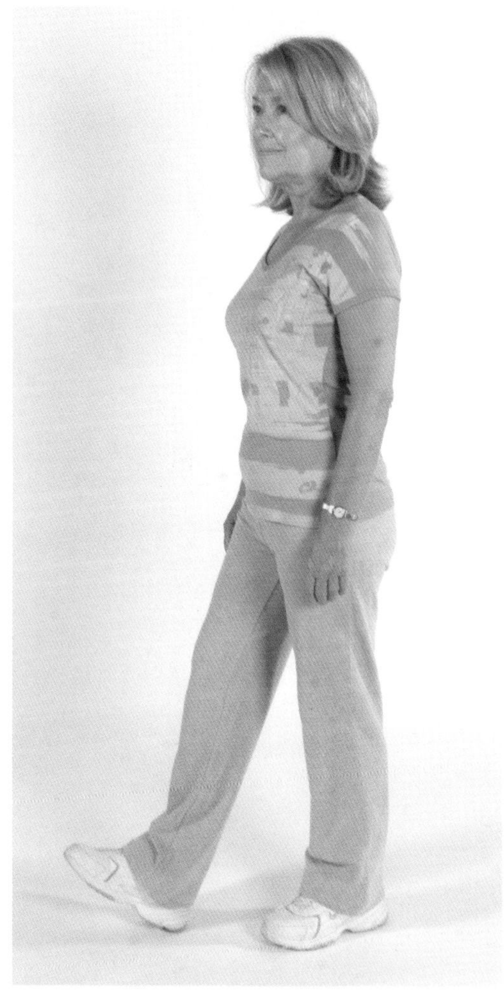

Heel–toe standing is an excellent balance exercise because it involves holding your balance midway in the stance. It is not about taking steps but about keeping your body balanced with one foot in front of the other.

heel–toe walking

In this exercise you move forward, maintaining your heel–toe stance.

- Hold on to a bench or rail for support
- Move forward slowly by placing one foot in front of the other. Keep your feet directly in line with each other
- Take 5 to 10 steps forward

AN EASIER START

- If you find this hard at first, just take 2 to 3 steps then build up to 5 steps

UPGRADE

- Take 5 to 10 steps forward then take 5 to 10 steps back
- Repeat four times

AS YOU PROGRESS

- Hold on to the bench with one finger
- Don't hold on
- Increase the number of times you walk forward and back
- Try each step with your eyes closed

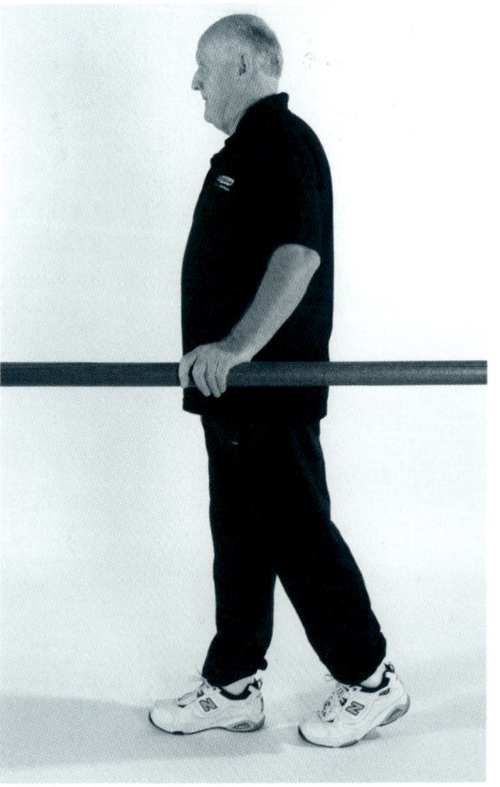

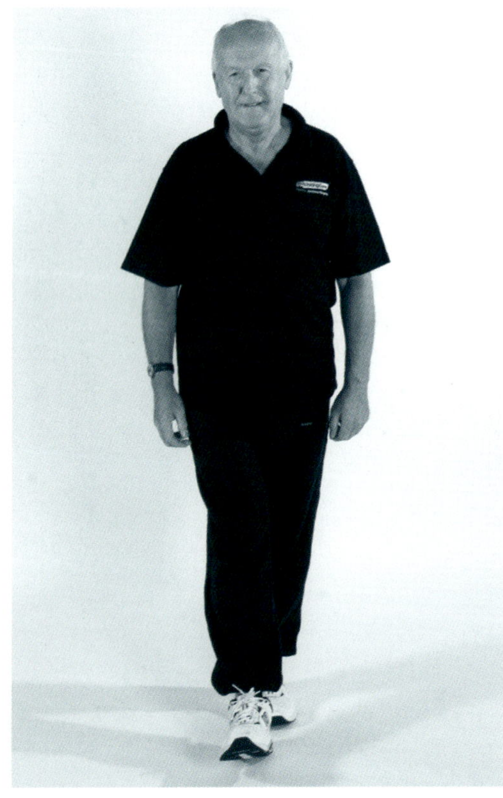

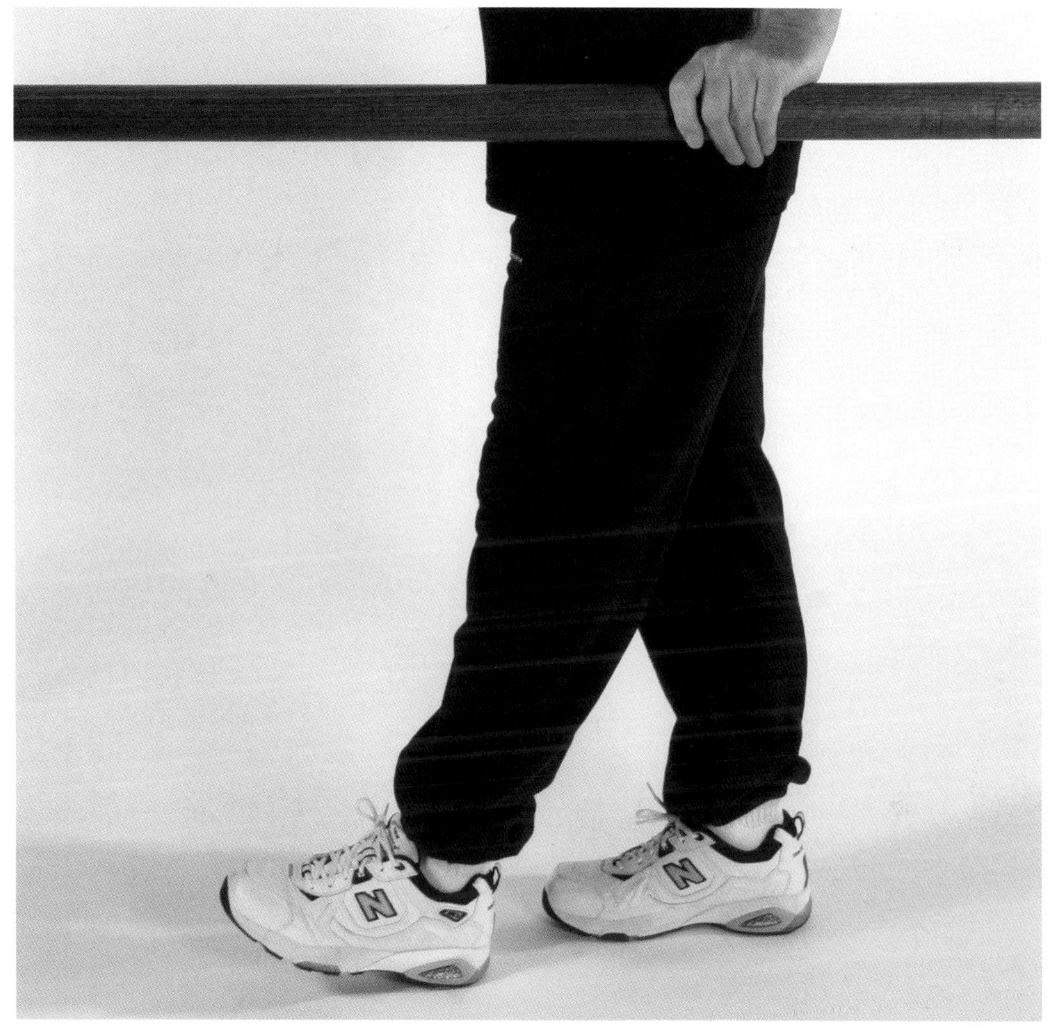

meet Marjorie Marjorie baby sits her grandchildren each week. One week she fell when she tripped over the toys that the children had left lying around. When she started the balance routine, Marjorie was surprised to find how difficult it was for her to stand in a "heel-to-toe" position. She had never thought about her balance before, let alone that she could do something to improve it. After doing the balance exercises for a little while, she found she was starting to weave her way around the toys much better.

finding your toppling point

In this exercise you become more aware of how it feels when you shift your weight. The idea is to find the point just before you overbalance and to hold this position for as long as possible.

- Stand tall with your hands by your sides and your feet shoulder width apart
- Lean to one side as far as possible, shifting your weight onto one foot. Keep your body straight and avoid bending at the waist
- Hold the pose for 15 seconds
- Repeat to the other side

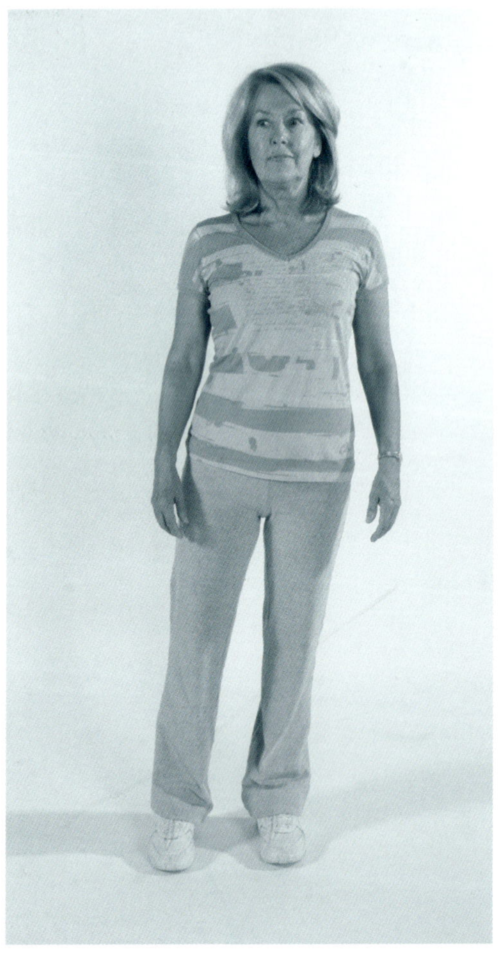

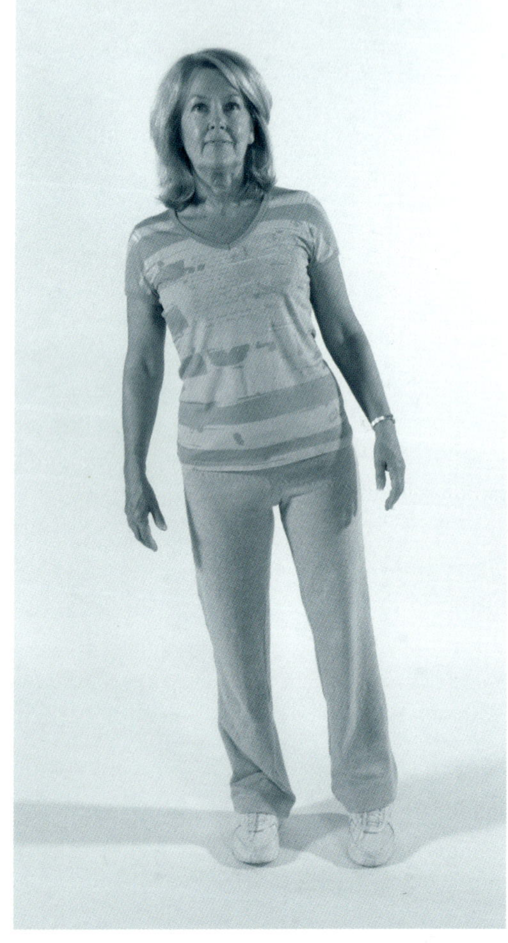

AS YOU PROGRESS

- Keep your feet closer together as you shift your weight
- Keep your feet closer together and your eyes closed

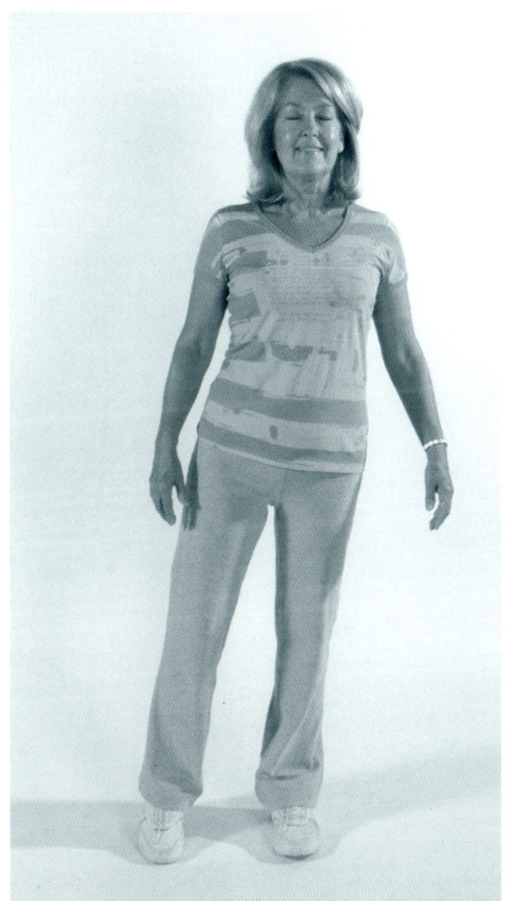

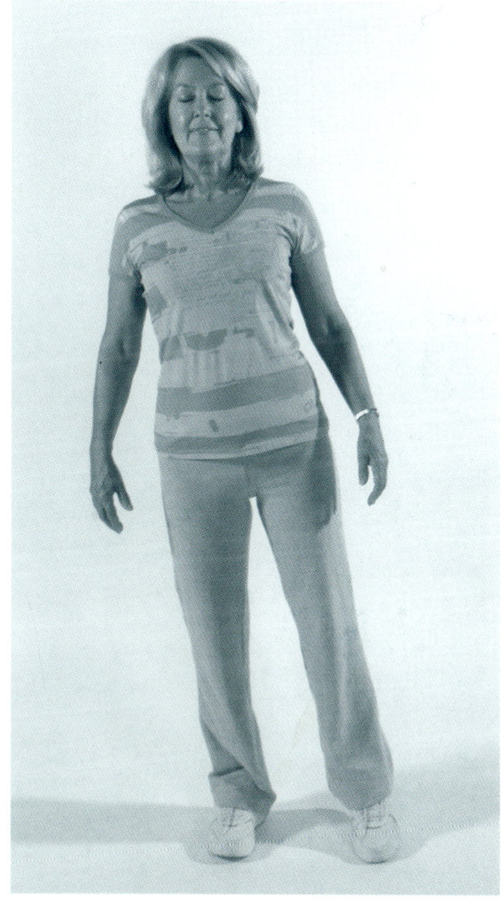

heel walking

This exercise is great for stretching and strengthening your ankles. It also improves your control when you walk.

- Hold on to a rail, bench, table or wall for support as you walk
- Stand tall and walk on your heels. Keep your toes off the floor as you walk
- Take 10 steps forward

Keep your toes off the floor as you walk

UPGRADE

- Increase the number of heel walks you do and the distance you walk

AS YOU PROGRESS

- Use just a finger to guide you
- Don't hold on

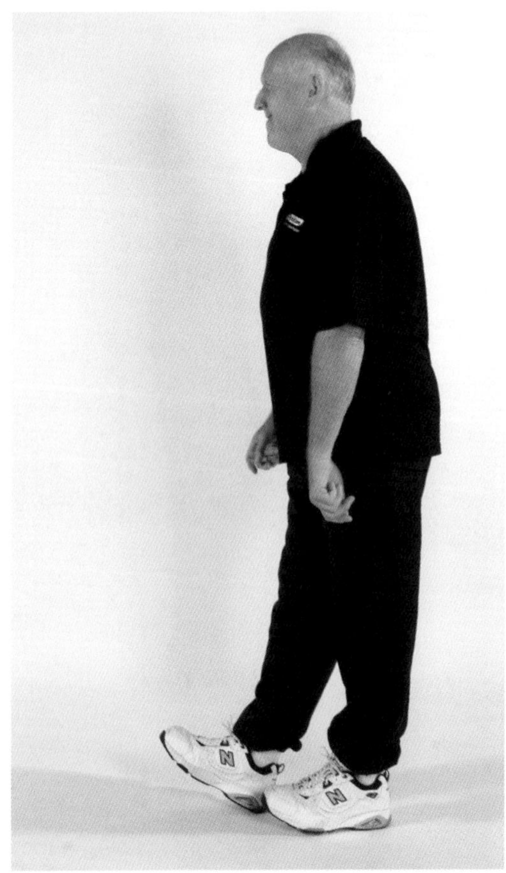

sideways walking

Do this exercise during your daily activities, such as whenever you walk down the hall to go to the front door.

- Stand tall with your feet hip distance apart and place your hands on your hips
- Take 10 steps to the right, then pause
- Take 10 steps to the left, then pause
- Repeat sequence

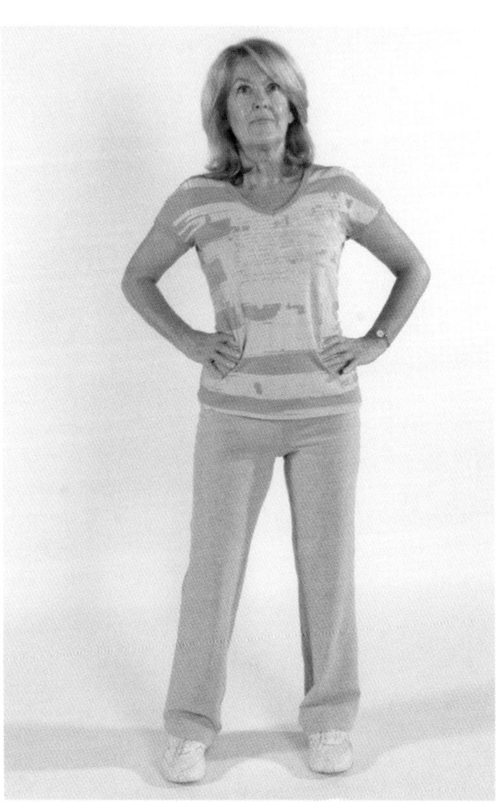

AN EASIER START

- Take 3 steps to each side
- Slowly increase the number of steps as your confidence builds

UPGRADE

- Start with 10 small steps then progress to 10 longer steps
- Take 10 slow steps to the right and 10 slow steps to the left without pausing

AS YOU PROGRESS

- Increase the number of repetitions until you are doing 10 steps four times to each side, with small breaks in between

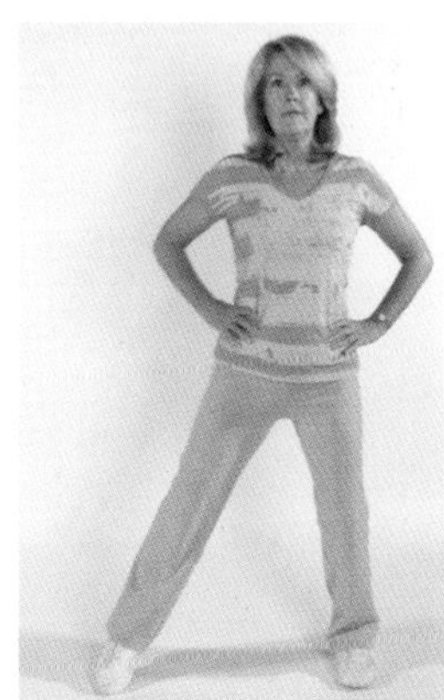

Do not do this exercise too quickly. Keep your head up, your back straight and tall, and try not to look at your feet as you step. This ensures that you are testing your balance.

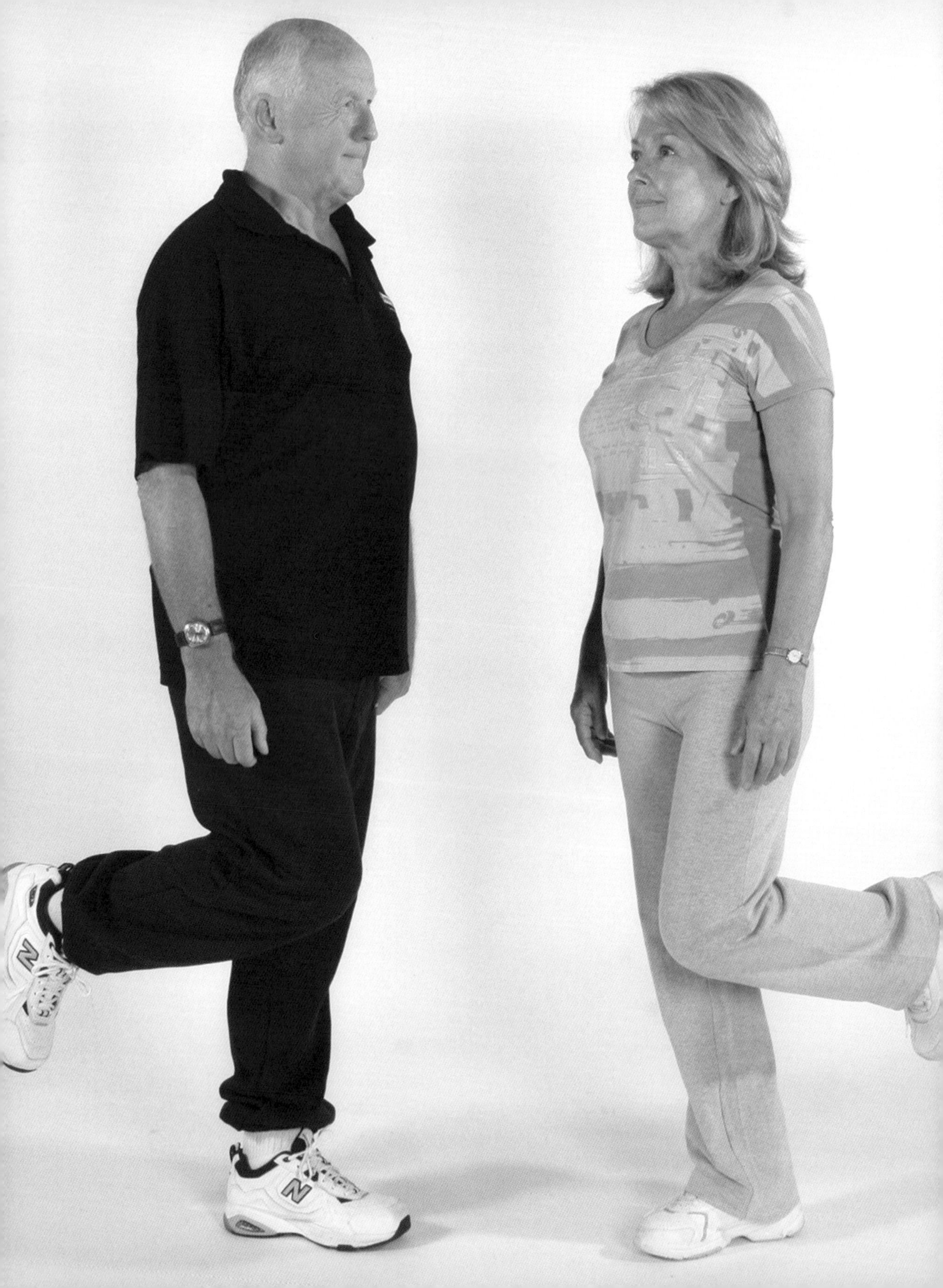

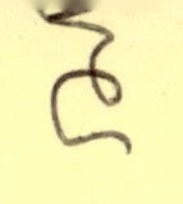

extending your balance practice

Once you have mastered these exercises, add additional balance routines to keep up your interest and extend the challenge.

TRY:

- standing on one leg
- walking then turning
- walking as you step over obstacles
- toe walking as well as heel walking

TO KEEP IMPROVING YOUR BALANCE:

- Use less hand support. Start each exercise holding on to a chair, table, rail or bench. As you improve you can reduce to a fingertip hold, then to no handhold. Each person's ability, no matter what age, is individual; everyone will start at a different balance level and increase at their own pace.
- Challenge your balance in different ways. For example, while standing, you can shift your body weight from one leg to another. This will test your balance because it involves shifting your centre of mass. The more you practise, the more your body learns to react to this changing posture with greater speed and skill.
- Keep increasing the difficulty of your balance routine.
- Challenge your balance further by doing the routines with your eyes closed. If you close your eyes while standing with your feet together or in tandem, you shut off sensory input, which makes it harder to control your muscles and to keep an upright posture. This is a great way to further challenge your balance, as long as you do it in a safe and controlled way, near a wall or sturdy chair.

CHAPTER 10

muscle strength

When you think about a champion runner, you visualise them with powerful legs that bulge with obvious muscle bulk. They walk with a strong stride and can tackle steps and stairs effortlessly. But you don't need to have the strength of an Olympic athlete to be able to improve the muscle bulk in your legs.

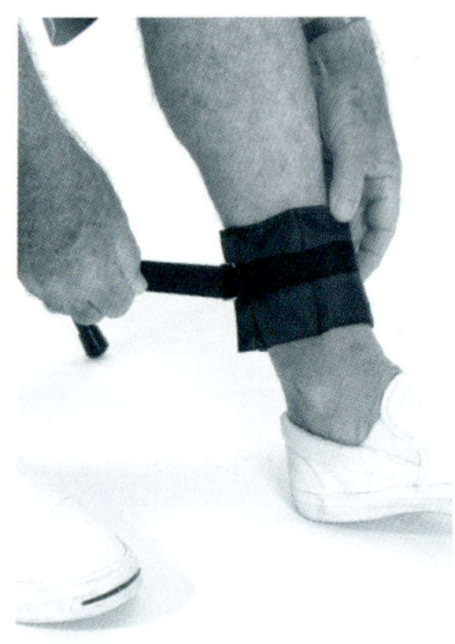

Putting a weight on your ankle will add resistance and increase your muscle strength

In fact, you can gain strength much more easily. The Olympian would need to train very hard to see even small gains in muscle strength; however, you will see good results in just two or three weeks if you do the following exercises.

Muscle fibre, and therefore muscle strength, begins to decrease after the age of 50, and decreases more rapidly after you reach 70 years of age. This can be associated with natural ageing processes but is more the result of a general reduction in physical activity. Weakness and disuse, however, are reversible at any age. Even people in their nineties can increase muscle strength by progressive strength training.

Slow change over time

Often we don't notice the loss of strength that occurs slowly over time. When James (see page 31) started to really reflect on the causes of his falls, he discovered that the changes in his body had been so subtle and gradual, he hadn't noticed them. Although he was still active and rushing about, he was starting to do a lot less than he used to. Sometimes it is easy to notice a significant weakness, especially after you have been sick or after long periods of inactivity. You might get out of bed one day and notice your legs feel

Weakness and disuse are reversible at any age. Even people in their nineties can increase muscle strength by progressive strength training.

like jelly. Strength can easily be lost like this, but with a bit of time and effort, you can also regain it.

Why improve your strength?

In a general sense, you exercise to:

- prevent falling
- compensate for biological ageing changes
- reverse the effects of muscle that has weakened through disuse
- cope with chronic disability or disease
- improve mobility
- make your body look aesthetically pleasing
- give yourself a general sense of wellbeing.

More specifically, if you increase your strength you will be able to:

- regain control better when you trip on something
- stop shuffling your feet
- feel confident enough to heel–toe walk
- make your stride stronger and longer.

If you keep these points in mind and practise positive self-talk about them, you will become more and more confident about your mobility and this in turn will reduce your falls risk.

meet Norma After doing the strength exercises for a few weeks, Norma noticed how much easier it was for her to get out of the seat at the theatre. She didn't have to wait for the lights to come on and her friend to help her. Her friend commented on the difference. Noticing little things like this helped build her confidence so she could continue her old lifestyle with a new awareness of falls risks, but also without worrying about it.

Strength training is about moving against resistance.

How to improve your strength

First, let's have a look at how muscles grow. Muscles are made of long, thin cells, grouped into strands called muscle fibres. These fibres are bundled tightly together, making up the muscle itself, like the fibres of a piece of rope. When muscles resist against a force, the fibres strain. Then, while you rest, your body repairs these tiny stresses. In doing so, the body overcompensates, making the fibres even stronger than they were before. This is how resistance exercise increases your strength.

So strength training is about moving against resistance. The resistance in your exercises comes from the weight of your body and limbs and, for some exercises, from the gradual inclusion of using small weights.

Add weights to get results

For best results, buy a set of ankle cuff weights that can be strapped to your ankle with a Velcro strap. You can get ankle cuff weights from some sporting stores, physiotherapy departments, specialised therapy suppliers and gymnasium equipment

meet Alan Alan, a rally car driver, was cynical about the exercises at first, saying he did not think they could possibly work because they looked too simple. However, he persevered with them. By the second week, he noticed for the first time in a long time that he was able to stand with confidence to put on his trousers. Other rally club members noticed how much better he was walking, and this made him feel more confident. It also made him more positive about the effectiveness of the exercises, which he resolved to keep doing.

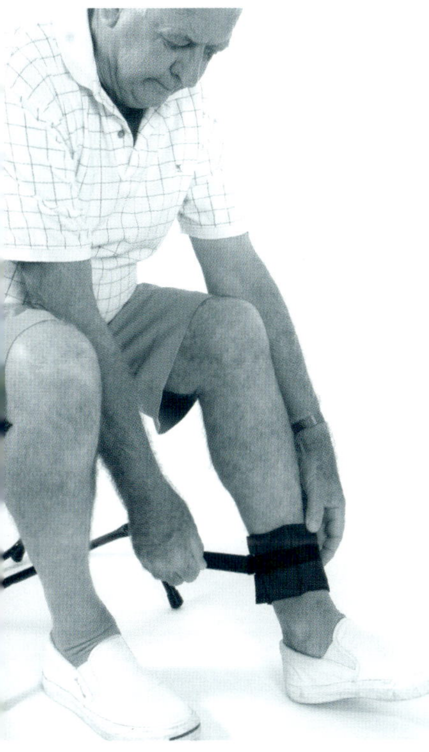

You can tighten the Velcro strap on the weight so that it fits snugly around your ankle

The body needs time to rebuild the muscles before you exercise them again.

suppliers. There are also some websites, such as www.australianbarbellco.com, where you can order cuffs and weights online. These websites sometimes give the local retail suppliers, which will be cheaper than paying for postage. If you sew, you could try making your own ankle cuff weight with pouches so you can insert heavier weights as you progress.

Regular practice

To make sure that your muscles continue to grow, you must do the exercises on a regular basis, three days each week. To make this happen, incorporate them into your weekly routine, making specific decisions about when you'll do them. Even write down a schedule so you remember. Copy the chart on page 156 every week and tick off each session as you complete it. This will help get you into the habit of doing your exercises and will become a personal record of your achievement. Keep up a chart for at least 7 to 12 weeks, longer if it helps.

Keep in mind that the body needs time to rebuild the muscles before you exercise them again, so rest the muscles on alternate days when doing intensive muscle-strength training. Avoid doing the exercises two days in a row.

Slow and deliberate movements

When you are doing the exercises, pause slightly between each one to allow the fibres to replenish their oxygen. Do each movement slowly and deliberately, concentrating on trying to feel the tension in your muscles. The only way you will load your muscles and gain strength is to focus on the exercises properly. Starting strength training is like starting to play a new game or sport—you work out your personal starting level and you slowly progress from there.

You may experience some muscle soreness when you first start training. This is a natural part of muscle strengthening. It will lessen and disappear as you train regularly. If you experience pain, you may need to talk to your doctor or physiotherapist. If you get pain from one particular exercise, talk to your physiotherapist about it. They can help you work out the problem, and adapt the exercise for your level.

Do each movement slowly and deliberately, concentrating on trying to feel the tension in your muscles.

Weights and repetitions

For the first week, we suggest you do the exercises without wearing any weights. When starting out, your own body weight will provide enough resistance. To gain strength and muscle mass from the knee and hip exercises, you will need to add a weight around your ankle. Start with 0.5-kilogram weights and progress to heavier weights as you get stronger. Also increase the number of times you repeat each move. Try to do 8 to 15 repetitions for each leg. If you can't manage at least 8 repetitions, the weight is too heavy. Weight lifting has enormous benefits for muscle, bone and ligaments as well as joint pain.

The exercises

The following strength-building exercises are simple but effective. When they are combined with the balance exercises, they reduce the risk of falls. They have been chosen specifically because they strengthen your ankles, knees and hips. These are the joints that really need to be strengthened to prevent falling.

You're likely to feel stronger and more able after just a few weeks of doing the muscle-strengthening exercises

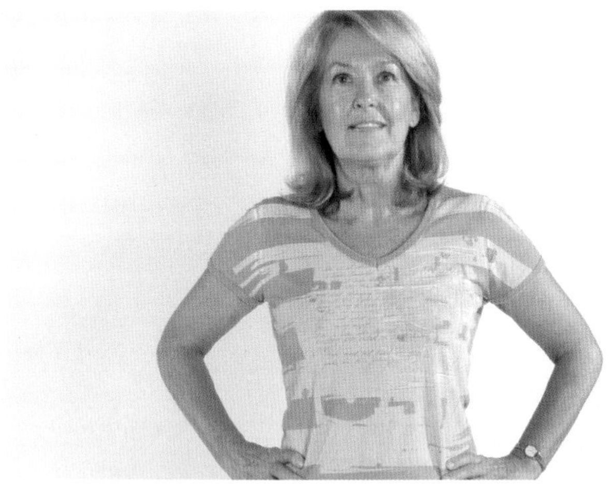

Often people don't believe in the exercises at first—especially men, who tend to want something a bit more sophisticated or intensive. But unlike balance, which can take a while to have clearly observable improvements, most people notice and comment that they feel stronger and more able after just a few weeks of doing dedicated strength exercises.

However, for the exercises to work, you have to keep them up. Chapter 11 suggests some different strategies to try when you experience a "relapse" and have difficulty maintaining your exercise routine. Plan ahead now for these times—they happen to us all. And remember, "if you don't use it, you lose it".

The muscle-strengthening exercises are:

- sit-to-stand slowly
- straight-leg raise
- hip-strengthening side raise
- calf raise

These four strength exercises, along with the five balance exercises, are the minimum we recommend you do to reduce your chances of having a fall.

THE MUSCLE-STRENGTHENING ROUTINE

These exercises are simple but effective. Once you have mastered each sequence at the simplest level, progress to a level that is "hard" to do. Once this level becomes not so hard, move directly up to the next level. As your strength improves, keep progressing.

sit-to-stand slowly

This exercise should be done slowly to challenge balance and gain maximum strength at the same time. The more slowly you go, the better it works because the muscles work harder.

- Sit on a chair
- Line up your feet so they are behind your knees
- Lean forward over your knees
- Push off from the chair with your hands and stand up slowly
- Hold your standing position for 5 seconds
- Repeat once

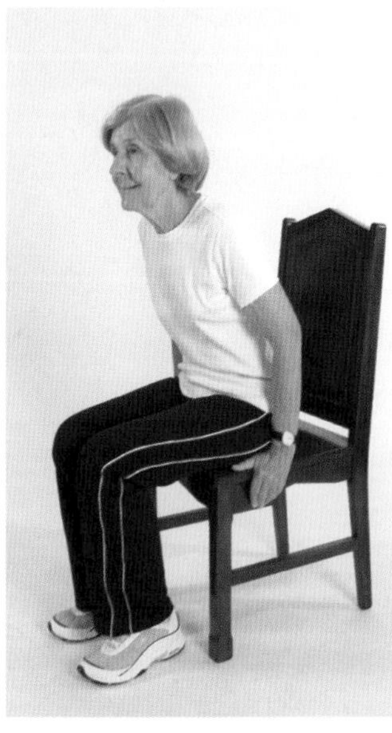
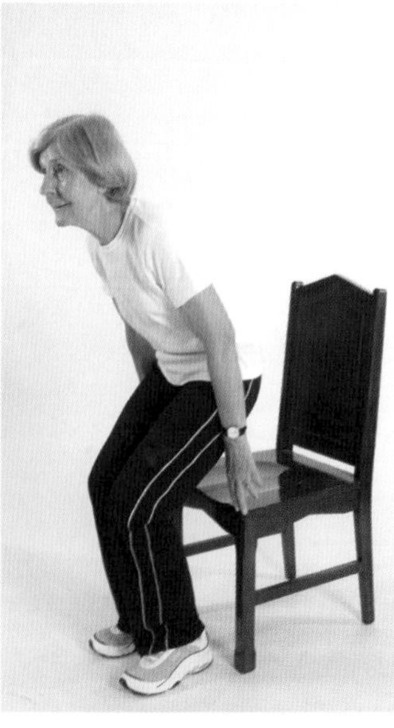
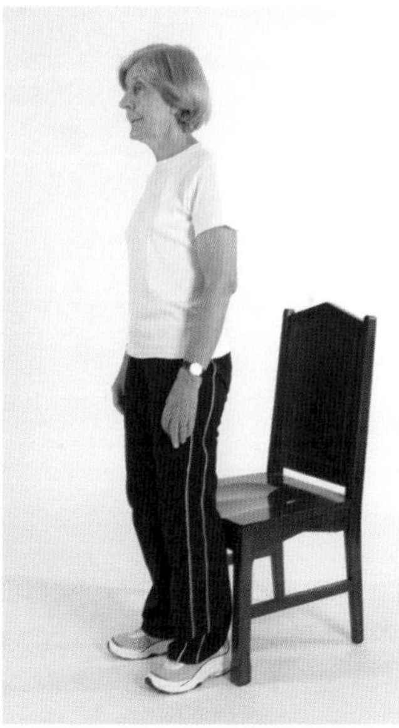

AN EASIER START

- Hold on to the sides of the chair for extra support

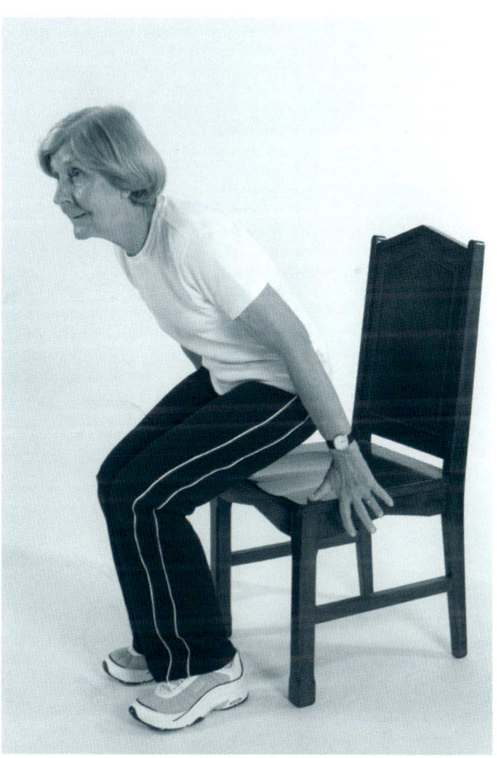

UPGRADE

- Stand up without pushing off with your hands
- Stand up more slowly
- Increase repetitions. Start with 5 repetitions, then increase to 10
- Further increase the number of repetitions as required

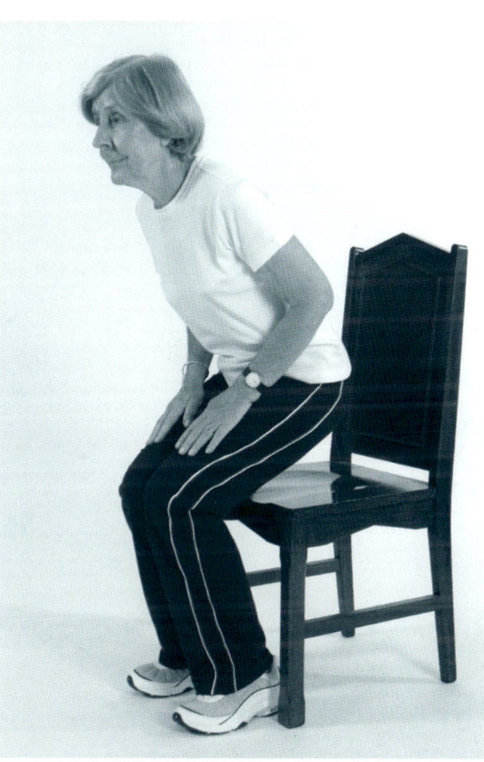

KEEP IN MIND

- Lean forward with your feet slightly apart
- Keep your shoulders over your hips
- Keep your head up and look forward

straight-leg raise

This is one of the main exercises in the program, and the most important for walking, climbing and other activities. Strong knees will help you regain control if you do trip.

- Strap a weight on to your ankle
- Sit on a chair with your back well supported
- Straighten your leg. Hold for 5 seconds.
- Lower your leg
- Repeat five times with your right leg then your left leg

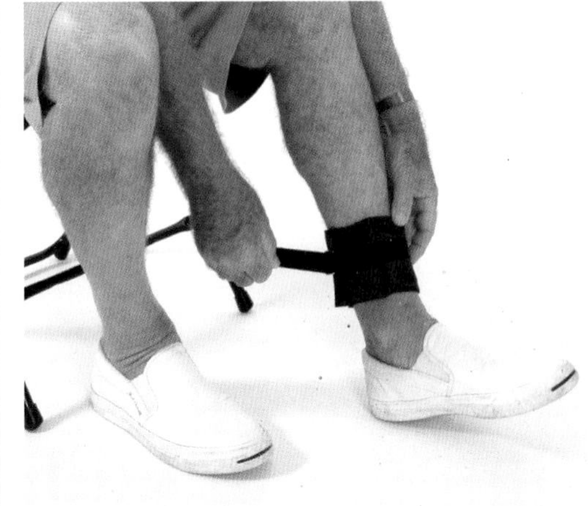

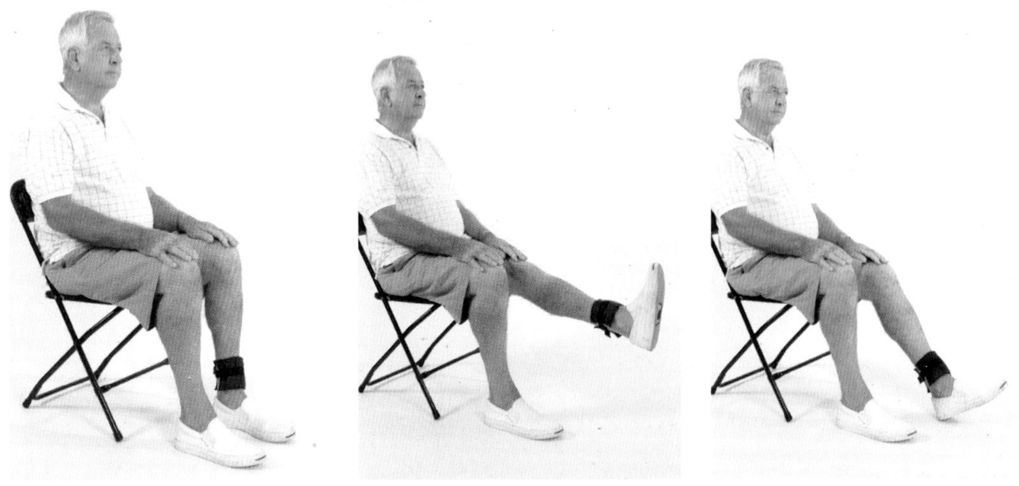

AN EASIER START

- Don't use any ankle weights
- If you continue to have problems with your knees or can't do this exercise after several weeks, ask your doctor for a physiotherapy consultation, and they will suggest alterations or alternatives

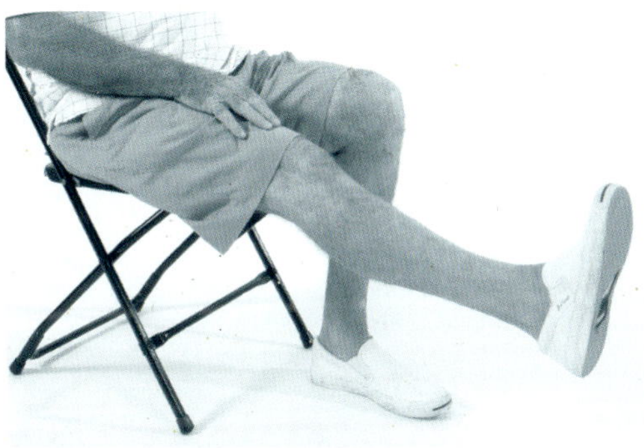

UPGRADE

- Increase repetitions to 10 and beyond
- Progressively increase the weights. Start with a 0.5-kilogram weight and work your way up
- Keep training at a level that is hard to do

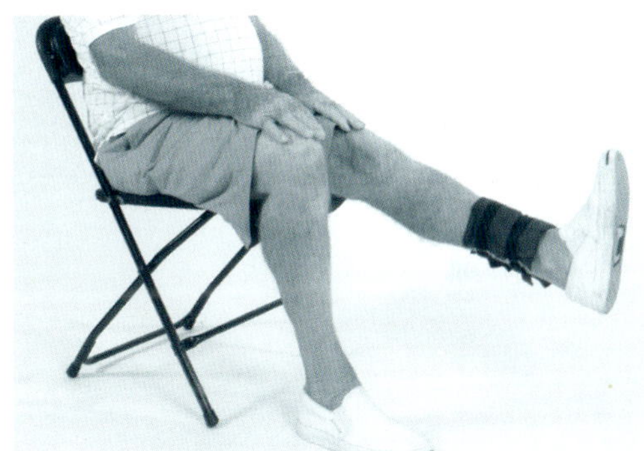

KEEP IN MIND

- You don't need to fully extend your knee to get benefit from this exercise, nor do you need to fully flex your ankle. Full extension of your knee will exercise extra muscles but it is not essential
- Make sure you lift your leg *slowly* so that you avoid the influence of momentum as much as possible. Doing the exercises quickly achieves far less; it might be easier but it reduces the resistance on your muscles

meet Helen Although Helen was keen to get into the balance and strength training, she had a lot of trouble with the exercises. Because of her sore back, she was at first concerned that she wouldn't be able to do them at all. But with the help of her physiotherapist, Helen toned down the exercises so that she could do them without hurting her back as much. Over time, as she became fitter and her back healed, the exercises were easier for her, so she gradually stepped up their intensity until she could do them without adaptation.

hip-strengthening side raise

This is an excellent exercise for building strong hips. Strong hips mean better control and easier walking and climbing.

- Put on the ankle cuff weights
- Hold on to a support such as a wall, rail, chair or bench with your right arm and keep your body straight and tall
- Lift the left leg out to the side then lower it in again
- Repeat five to ten times
- Turn around and repeat with the right leg

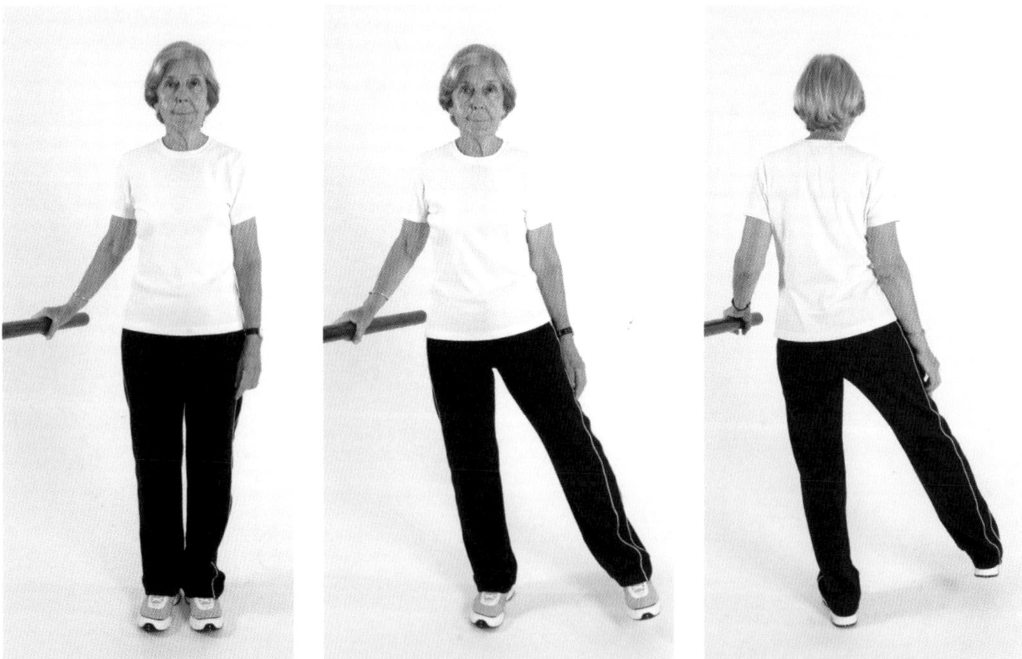

Learn the correct moves first without wearing a weight. Put on the weights as soon as possible and keep progressing

AN EASIER START

- Shift your weight onto your weight-bearing leg first, before you raise the other leg
- If you have back problems, lie sideways on a bed, then do the exercise

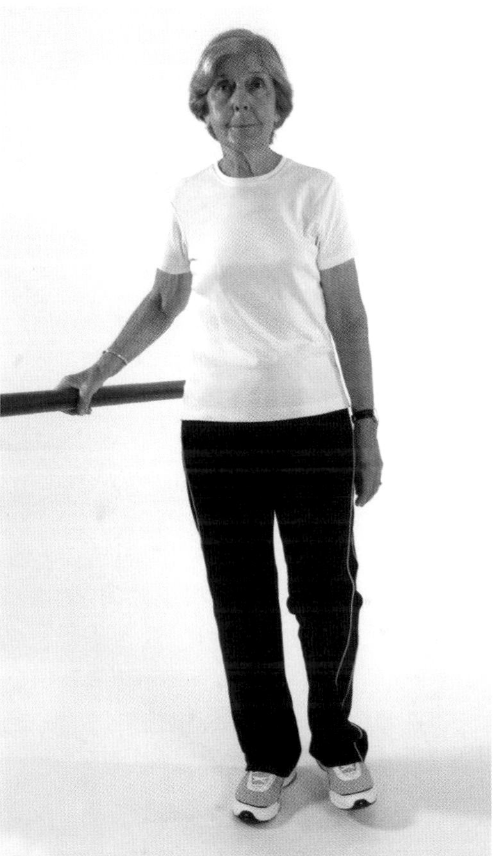

UPGRADE

- Increase to 10 repetitions
- Progressively increase the heaviness of the weight

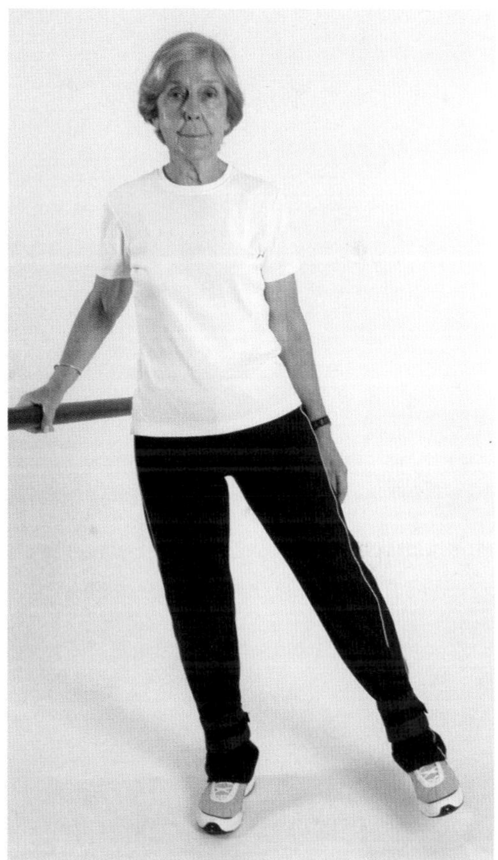

KEEP IN MIND

- Under normal circumstances, you need to do this exercise standing upright with your back straight
- Try practising in front of a mirror. This makes it easier to keep an upright posture.
- Lift your leg slowly to avoid momentum

calf raise

This exercise combines ankle strengthening and balance, and is very important for strength and control in heel–toe walking. It also strengthens your calves and helps you avoid the dangerous "shuffle walking".

- Stand up tall near a wall or chair for support with your feet shoulder width apart
- Hold on to your support with both your hands
- Stand on your toes
- Lower your heels to the ground
- Repeat 5 to 10 times slowly

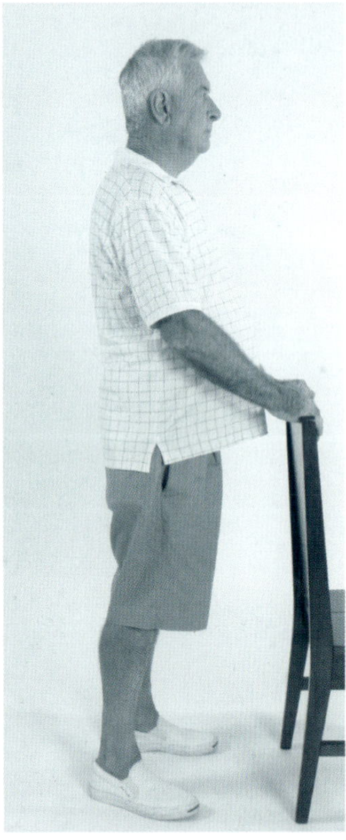
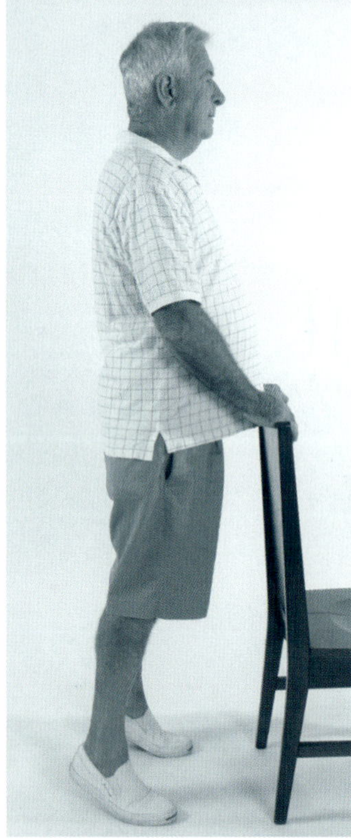
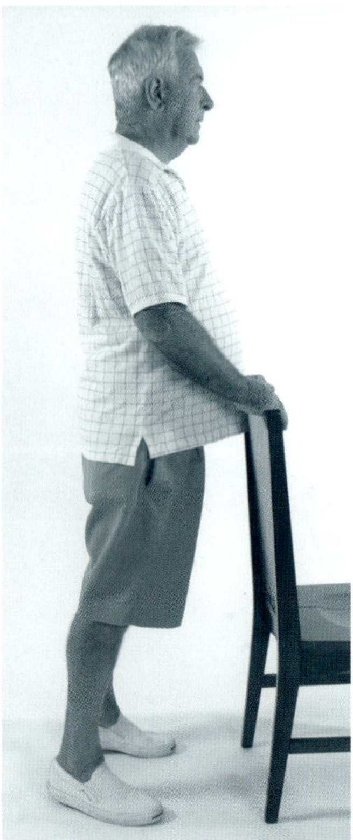

UPGRADE

- Increase to 20 repetitions
- Reduce hand support to a finger, then to none

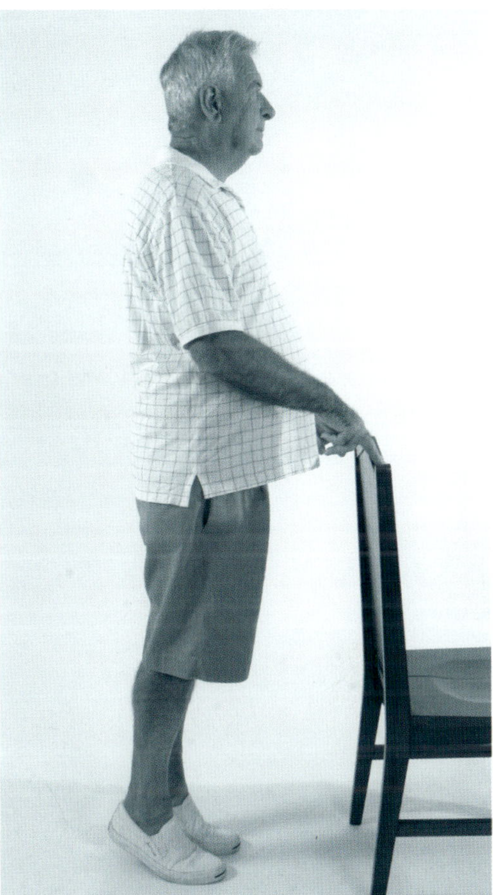

For more detailed or prescriptive exercise programs, ask your physiotherapist or exercise instructor.

other exercises

There are other strength exercises that you can add to your routine later for variety. These include:

- standing on one leg and flexing your knee
- climbing the stairs slowly

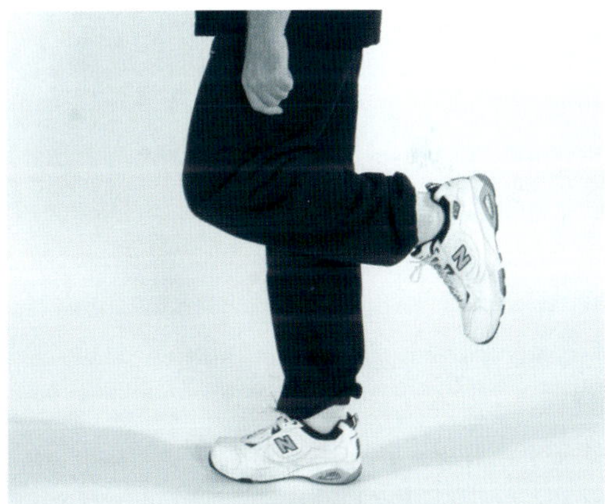

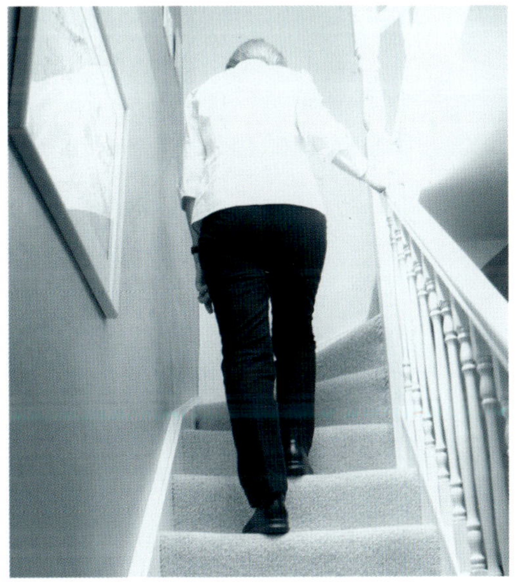

getting your exercise routine in place

It's important to get into a routine of doing both your balance and strength exercise regularly. So plan which days of the week you will do the exercises.

CONSIDER THESE QUESTIONS:

- Are you a morning or evening person?
- When does it suit you to do the exercises?
- What will help you to remember to do them?

TO GET THE BEST RESULTS:

- Remember, for the best results, do each exercise three to four times a week. It's better to avoid using the weights on consecutive days as your muscles need time to recover between sessions.
- Create a weekly Exercise Record Chart. There's one on page 156 you can copy and use. Tick off the exercises as you do them each day.
- "Breaking through barriers to exercise" on page 90 gives you more practical ideas to help get you started.

You can do your leg raises while you are watching TV

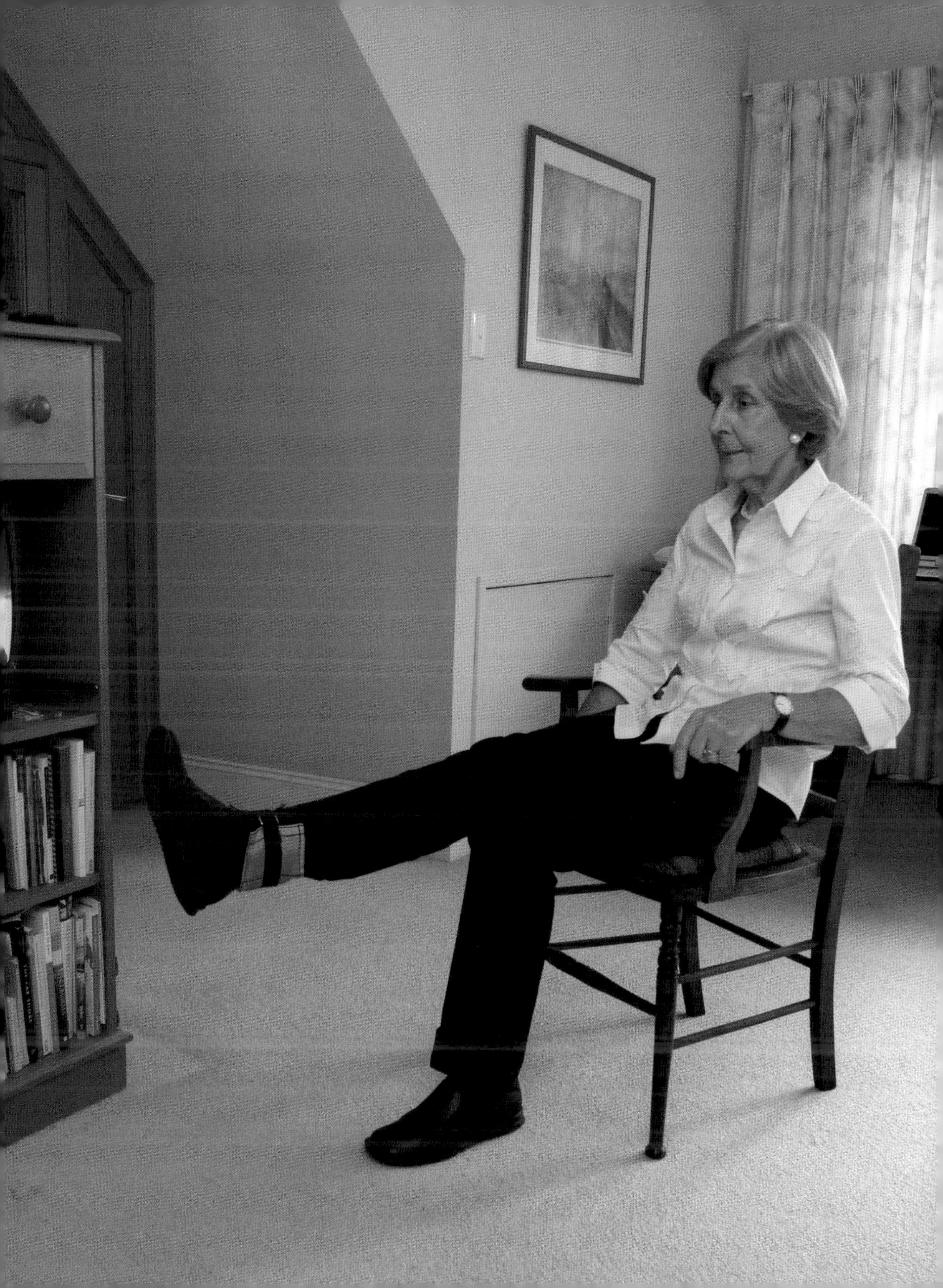

CHAPTER 11

making exercise count

The exercises in chapters 9 and 10 will help you with your balance and strength, help you walk with a strong heel–toe stride and help reduce your risk of falling when you are doing what you need to during the day. If you do the exercises regularly, they will also get you ready for more physical activity in general.

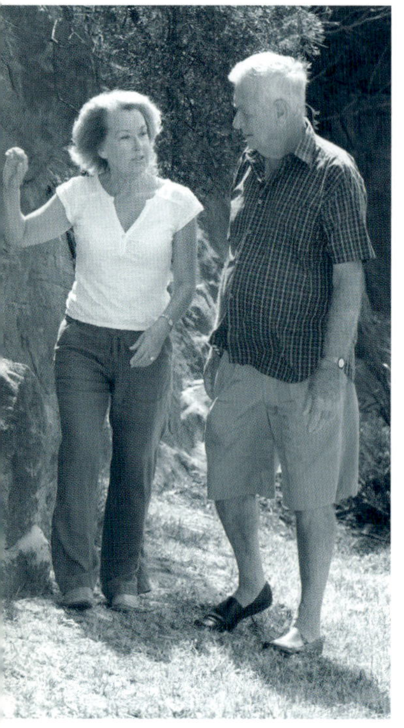

If you keep up the balance and strength training, you will find walking easier and a lot more pleasurable

Increasing your physical activity

Walking is a great place to start. If you do the balance and strength exercises outlined and keep them up, you will find walking easier and a lot more pleasurable.

Walking is good for your health but a fear of falling often stops people from venturing out. To walk well with a firm heel–toe stride, you need to be strong, and you need to have the confidence to know that your balance is good enough to cope with uneven ground, and gutters and steps.

As you work through the next chapters, you will get an understanding of the broader range of contributors to a fall, which will empower you to know how to deal with them. You will find that exercise is the cornerstone of dealing with many of these factors.

Some research has shown the benefits of Tai Chi in improving balance and reducing falls, so this could be something worth considering. Once you feel stronger and your balance is better, think about joining a community class for general exercise. However, we strongly recommend you continue our set of balance and strength exercises to keep your fall risk down.

"I am more conscious of the spring in my step. I say to myself "heel–toe, heel–toe" as I walk. Now I have a sense of control and feel more confident."

MARYJANE

As your strength and balance improves, think of how you can become more active in your daily and weekly routine, both at home and when you are out in your local community. Here are some examples, but find ways that will work for you.

- get up to change the TV channel instead of using the remote control
- cross the road at the traffic lights rather than using the most direct route
- walk to the shops instead of driving
- walk to the local post box to post a letter instead of driving to the post office
- go and say hello to the neighbours instead of using the phone
- get off the bus a few stops early and walk the rest of the way home
- take the stairs instead of the lift or escalator
- when you have visitors, suggest a walk outside before or after having a meal
- carry the groceries yourself instead of getting help
- do some gardening (or some other outside moderate physical activity) whenever the weather permits. Even half an hour is beneficial. The sun will give you vitamin D and help your muscles at the same time
- stand to do the ironing and folding the clothes.

meet Liz Liz is often busy babysitting and explained that she had really wanted to do the exercises so she could keep up with the kids. At first she didn't think she'd have the time to do the routines, but being better able to look after the kids once she'd started the exercises led her to even start doing them while looking after the kids. So she made the time. Her improved energy with the kids was the one thing that kept her motivated.

"When I got the weights I knew I was on the right track. You sort of think they are too easy [the exercises] then you suddenly find they work."

BILL

Make plans to do some of these things with a friend or family member. It's often easier to achieve your goal when you make a commitment with someone else.

Breaking through barriers to exercise

When you first start to introduce changes to your life, you are likely to come up against difficulties. Even if you go through the stages of making a plan, breaking it down into small manageable steps and setting realistic goals, there will still be barriers that could hinder your success. If you don't recognise and deal with these barriers, they can stop you achieving your goals and leave you at risk.

In Part 2 we looked at barriers in general and looked at how to recognise, avoid and negotiate them. However, dealing with barriers is especially relevant when you are trying to establish an exercise routine. As you know by now, exercises that build balance and strength form the core of any sincere attempt at falls reduction. And yet, because of the time and effort required to do them properly and regularly, they can also be the easiest part to leave out.

Many barriers can prevent you from starting and sustaining an exercise routine. These include:

- accepting weakness and poor balance as an inevitable part of ageing
- not having enough time (or thinking that you don't)
- not understanding the need for exercise and how it helps you
- not understanding how to do all of the exercises properly
- lacking confidence or having a fear of falling during the exercises

- having a fear of pain
- forgetting to do the exercises
- doing too much too quickly
- not having a planned program with gradual increases, which leads to being overwhelmed or feeling defeated
- not stopping to think about how much better you feel and how much easier it is to do some things.

So far, we've explained how to do the exercises safely and how to work at your own level. We've looked at a number of myths that can prevent you from looking after yourself and so need to be challenged. We've emphasised the idea that the biggest hurdle as you age is to counteract the effects of disuse and inactivity. Remember, the reality is "if you don't use it, you lose it".

Only you can work out what your own barriers are ... and how you can overcome them.

But because these barriers are all so varied and personal, there is no single "correct" way to deal with them. You need to think about your own personality and lifestyle, and pool all the things that you have learnt to make your own judgements and decisions. Only you can work out what your own barriers are or will be, and how you can overcome them. However, while we can't tell you exactly what to do, we can suggest methods to help you break through your barriers.

The balance sheet

The best technique we found for exploring the pros and cons of regular exercise is the balance sheet. As we saw in Part 2, you can become more aware of your own motivations and hindrances by highlighting the advantages of exercise as well as the barriers. This helps you recognise and remember the benefits while weighing these up against the negatives—a balancing act of sorts, which can focus your thoughts on how to overcome any barriers you might face.

Another useful feature of the balance sheet is that it helps to pre-empt some of the barriers to exercising before you reach them, so that you can get the full benefit of the exercise as quickly as possible. It also provides an opportunity to explore some alternative decisions and their positive effects.

We recommend that you write up your own balance sheet with your own lists. However, the pros and cons on these pages are some that people have suggested to us from their own experience. When creating your sheet, the aim is to list as many good things you can think of about exercising and as many negative things . Don't be afraid if your ideas seem silly. It is the process of getting them out that is important. This process helps you recognise both the difficulties and the positive outcomes of starting an exercise routine, and of keeping it going over time, so you stay focused and are prepared for setbacks.

Pros

- allows you more freedom
- strengthens your legs
- makes you feel good
- stops you falling
- makes you feel you're doing something for yourself

meet Kevin Kevin, a retired professor, summed it up. He commented that almost all the cons could be grouped into either time or commitment issues. He observed that he had plenty of time and just needed the commitment, while others had the commitment but needed to make time.

> "After the third week of doing these balance and strength exercises I have improved and feel real good. I've even done some dancing—haven't done that for a long time."
> KEVIN

- lubricates joints
- allows you to go out more
- you're not so tired or sore all the time
- improves and maintains mobility
- improves whole body
- creates better balance, better control
- you feel like you're in control
- you can do more physically
- improves independence, not relying on others
- allows you to stay in your own home
- gets you going in the morning.

Cons

- you don't have not enough time
- they become too boring
- commitment you're not sure you want
- you're retired, sounds like work
- you don't have the energy
- another thing you have to do for your body
- you know you won't remember
- you're too busy
- you like to do things with friends
- they might hurt your back
- they might be hard on your joints
- they make you feel a bit tight
- they're hard to fit in
- you're not sure if they will work.

Try this

Look at the lists of pros and cons on these pages. Which ones apply to you? Can you add any?

Think about the positives of balance and strength training and the barriers. What could you do to tip the scales in a positive direction and overcome the barriers that you see ahead?

Rephrasing your thoughts

Sometimes dealing with a barrier is a matter of reframing it so it sounds more positive. For example, "I haven't got time to do the exercises, I don't have the energy" can be reframed as, "Often by doing the exercises, I get more energy anyway". Think about the way you approach your barriers. Are you setting up the problems negatively in your head? Are you focusing on what you think you can't do or what you believe you can?

If you focus on what you'll be getting out of the exercises ... you will want to overcome the barriers in your way.

Staying positive

In the list of "pros" on pages 92–3, it is clear that although "reducing the risk of falls" is certainly there, many of the positive things are more to do with how you think about yourself—about gaining a sense of freedom, achievement and confidence. It's not surprising really. After all, who doesn't want to feel better about themselves?

It's almost certain that you'll come up against some difficulty in setting up and continuing with your exercise routine. But if you focus on what you'll be getting out of the exercises, which will help motivate you to want to do them, then you will also want to overcome the barriers in your way. By developing a constructive attitude and using positive self-talk to motivate and reward yourself, the process of dealing with barriers won't seem like a chore, but more a personal challenge that will allow you to grow and feel great about yourself.

Another great way to feel good about your progress, even when it seems things are going wrong, is to talk to friends and relatives about it. Some people get embarrassed when they have to expose to others

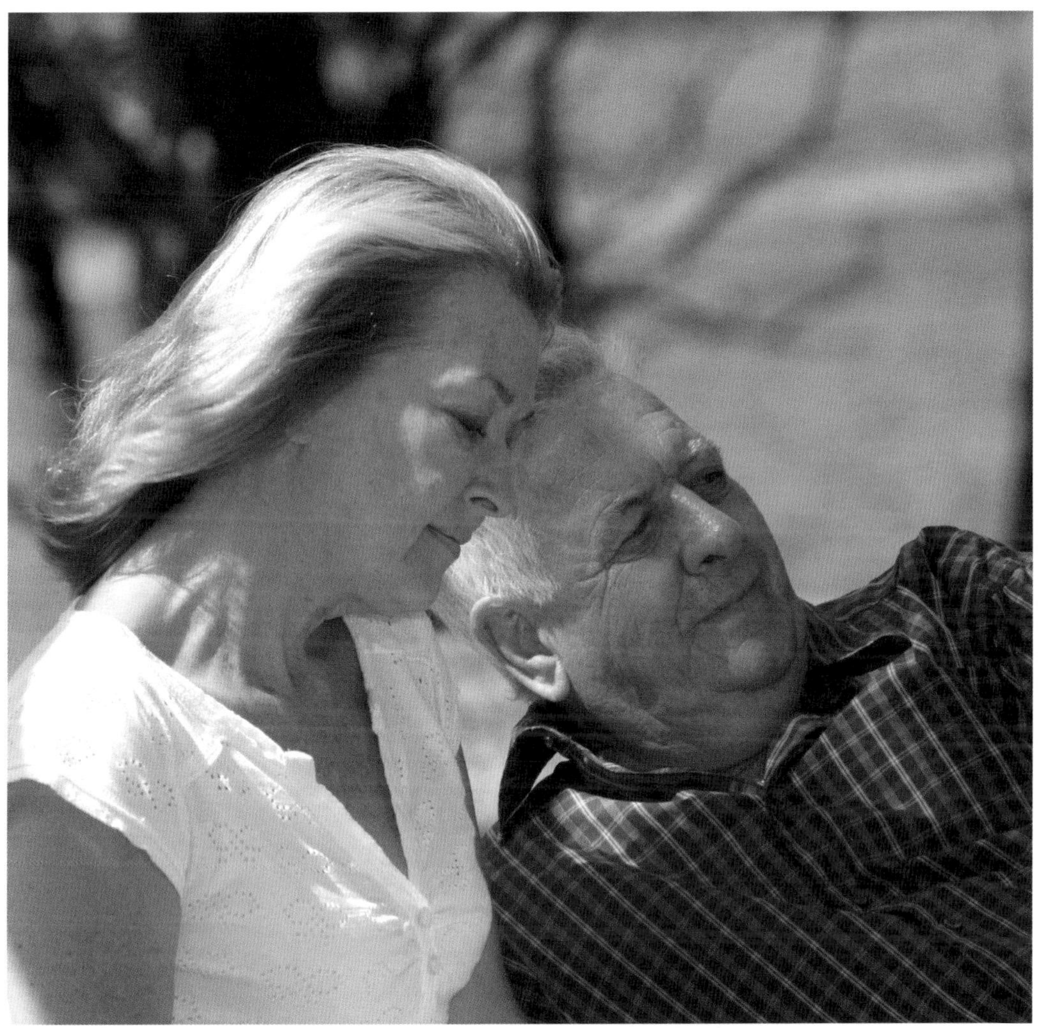

meet Rachel Rachel had arthritis and it was starting to cause her a lot of pain. She lived alone, which was always a great source of pride for her, and it seemed natural that these exercises were the best way for her to stay independent. So, rather than just giving up because of the pain, she slowly progressed with the exercises, keeping just below her pain threshold, and she rewarded herself with praise each week when she stuck to her routine. The fact that she was overcoming her pain became a source of pride in itself.

that they do these "silly" exercises. Finding the confidence to talk to others about them can be really affirming and give you a great boost of confidence to keep them up.

Other ideas

Copy the Exercise Record Chart on page 156 and tick off when you do each exercise. This helps you get into the habit of regular exercise and keeps you on track. This kind of monitoring can increase exercise activity by about 35 per cent—a really good outcome!

In our experience, the people who become committed to the exercises tend to find a particular time of the day when they can incorporate them into their daily routine. Others have found it easier to work them in as they go about their daily life, for example, doing the calf raises or heel–toe standing while on the telephone or waiting in line with the shopping trolley, sideways walking down the hall or to the front door, or doing leg raises while watching TV at night. We encourage you to do a portion of the exercises throughout the day if you feel like it, but remember that by the end the day, you do need to have done them all correctly.

"Doing the exercises is just like cleaning my teeth; it's become so normal to my life now."

HELEN

"Cuing" your memory with reminders works well for many people. If you always keep this book or your exercise chart in a particular spot, it becomes a trigger for remembering to do the exercises until they become a habit. Each time you see the book, it prompts your memory.

Dealing with relapse

If you lapse, try not to let it discourage you; just pick up again and return to your routine.

Once habits have been established, the most common barrier that people will face is a relapse—that is, having a break in the exercises and not starting again. Although a relapse is certainly not desirable, it's also not unusual. If you do lapse, try not to let it discourage you; just pick up again and return to your routine. In fact, having the relapse experience can provide an advantage. As you go through the experience and learn from it, you will be in a better place to stop it from happening again in the future.

A relapse often happens after a period of illness or holiday. One suggestion for avoiding this is to maintain the exercises over that period in a very modified form. It's much easier to build up from a little rather than none. In reality, most of us lapse into our old ways at some time, so make a commitment when you start your exercise routine to draw up an action plan to help you deal with a relapse if or when it happens.

To devise your relapse action plan:

1. Make a balance sheet listing the pros (what is good for me about doing these exercises) and the cons (what is not so good about doing these exercises, what could make it harder to start or keep doing them).
2. Think about your lists. Highlight the cons that potentially could cause you to relapse. Which cons could you change or be more positive about, to help you get started with your exercises and keep going? What in your list of pros can you focus on to help you to get started and keep going?

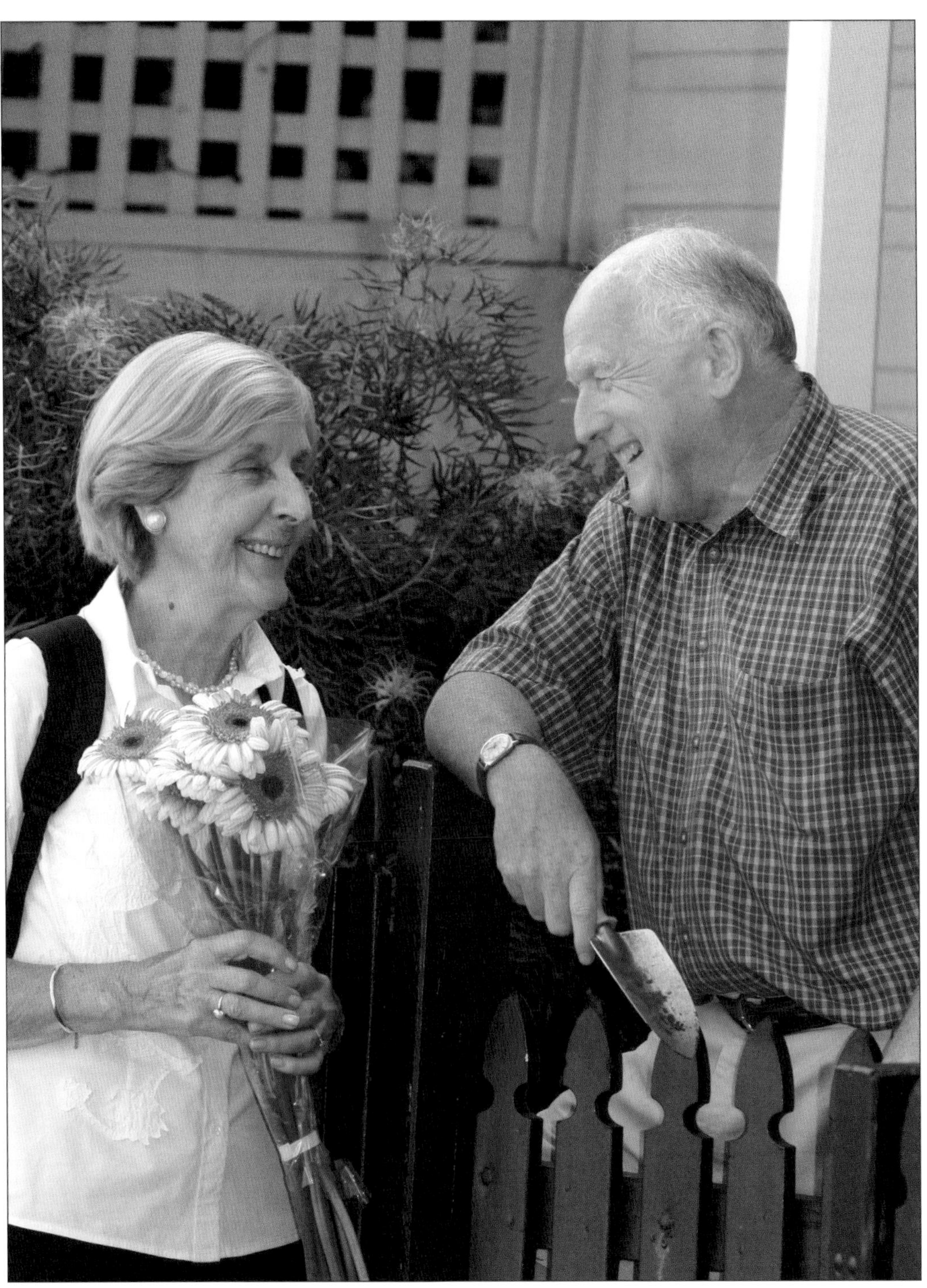

feeling safe at home and in your community

CHAPTER 12
home safety

There are often a number of contributing factors to a having a fall. In this chapter we aim to raise your awareness of some of the hazards that can cause falls at home. With more awareness, you'll be able to observe and identify hazards in your own environment, then start to think about how you can reduce your own risk.

Home hazards

We'll be identifying some of the most common home hazards. We'll help you to notice these hazards and give you some ideas for dealing with them before they cause a fall.

Often you don't see the hazards at home, such as clutter in walkways or dim lighting near stairs, because they are part of your everyday environment. We often don't recognise these things as a problem, even though they pose a risk. The hazard may be a habit or an unsafe pattern of thought, like using a chair to reach things in high cupboards. We are so used to doing things this way that we just don't think of them as hazardous. To change our thoughts, we need to pull our potentially hazardous actions into our consciousness for a while. Then we can change our behaviour to form new habits.

A closer look at hazards

When you think of the hazards in your environment and how to address them, use this question plan:

1. What is the hazard?
2. What can I do to change it?

meet Dorothy

Dorothy had asked her husband to cut back the camellia tree so that it didn't drop leaves on the front porch. It had also grown too large and was stopping the natural sunlight. The tree was a rare variety and her husband stubbornly resisted anything but a light trim. After a heavy hail storm Dorothy noticed its leaves on the front porch. She was in a hurry as she had to pick up the grandchildren from the railway station. Angrily, she grabbed the broom and started sweeping but she didn't realise that the broom and path were both wet. She turned and fell heavily, landing on her hip. As she lay on the porch, she thought, ironically, "I just finished putting elastic on the bottom of his pyjama pants to stop him tripping when he goes up and down the steps!"

THINK A MOMENT

- What do you think are the causes of Dorothy's fall?
- What can be done to prevent it happening again?

COMMENT

Preventing falls in and about your home is about making changes to your environment and to the way you do things within it. In Dorothy's situation, the tree needed severe pruning. Her husband needed to understand the risks if he left it unpruned. Attaching self-adhesive non-slip strips to step edges would make the steps safer. These are all changes to the environment that would make it safer. However, there are also behaviours that Dorothy could change to make this situation safer. Doing things quickly when you feel angry contributes to a risky situation. Being more aware of fall hazards can alert you to situations like slippery paths where you might be at more risk than usual.

3. Are there any barriers that will stop me making this change?
4. How do I keep the change to the hazard in place?

Most people think that most falls happen in the bathroom. But it's actually the place with the lowest incidence. In fact, 30 per cent of falls occur in living areas, 25 per cent in garages and outdoor areas, 20 per cent in bedrooms, 10 per cent in kitchens, 9 per cent on steps and stairs and only 6 per cent in bathrooms.

The following hazards cause the most falls at home:

- slippery surfaces
- obstacles in traffic ways
- poor lighting
- climbing and over reaching
- steps and stairs
- uneven, broken, loose or slippery pathways
- curled, loose or slippery floor mats
- unsuitable footwear
- a slippery bath, hazardous grab rail or no grab rail
- spills on the floor.

Most people think that most falls happen in the bathroom. But it's actually the place with the lowest incidence.

How to identify and deal with the hazards in your home

The following quiz is designed to make you more aware of the hazards around your own home that may cause you to fall. It should also guide your thoughts about making your home environment more safe. For each question, there can be more than one correct answer. Think about the option that best suits you.

home hazards quiz

For each scenario, ask yourself these four questions (remember there can be more than one correct answer):

- What do you do now?
- What should you do?
- What might be the barriers to doing this?
- What could you do to make it easier to keep it that way?

Tick the action(s) or habit(s) that would help prevent a fall. Place a cross next to the one(s) more likely to cause a fall.

1. IN THE BEDROOM:

- ❑ I let the bed clothes trail over the edge of the bed.
- ❑ I clear the clutter off the floor.
- ❑ I leave the cord from the television across the floor.
- ❑ I leave my shoes in the middle of the floor.

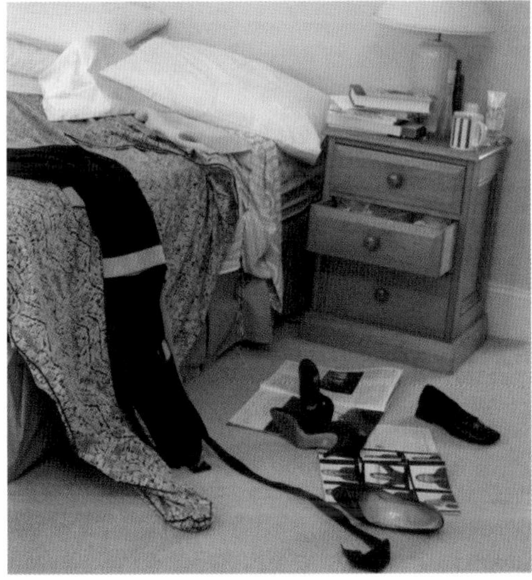

BEFORE: There are plenty of hazards in this familiar bedroom scene that could cause a fall

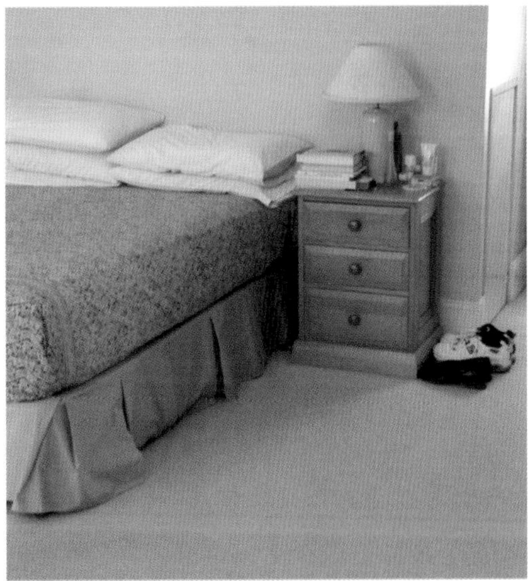

AFTER: Tidying the bed clothes and finding a new "spot" for the magazines and shoes will reduce your chances of falling

2. WHEN I HEAR THE TELEPHONE RING:

- ❑ I go as fast as I can in case they hang up.
- ❑ I check that the route to the phone is free of clutter.
- ❑ I move slowly and carefully.
- ❑ I leave a window open to hear the phone when I'm outside.
- ❑ I don't worry if I don't make it. I just press *10# to find out who the last caller was. (Note that the re-call code may differ between carriers and countries.)
- ❑ I have my cordless phone so I can answer it.

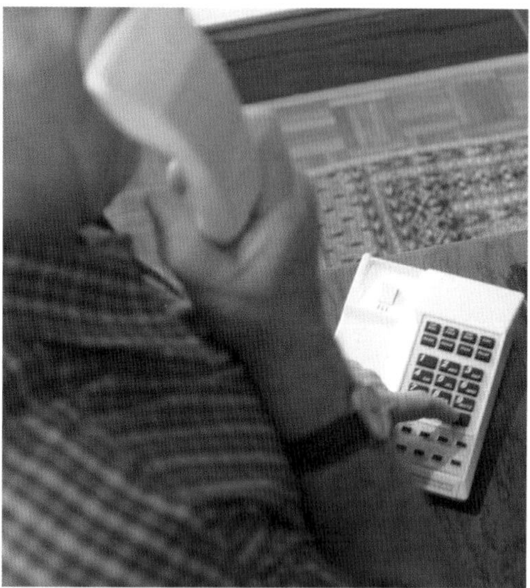

If you're not sure what the re-call code for your phone is, ask someone to show you how to use it so you don't have to rush in future

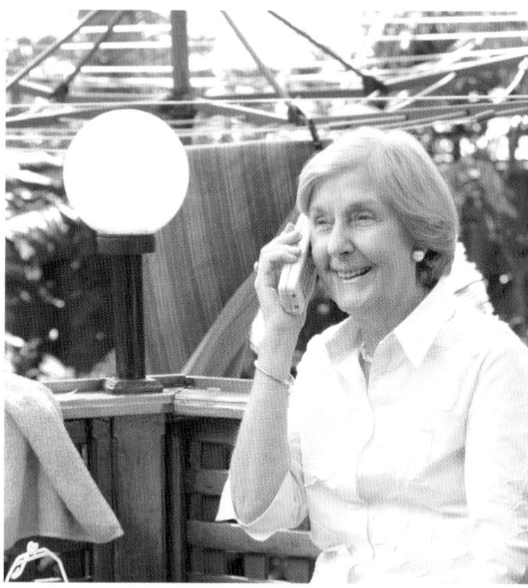

A cordless phone is really handy if you are outside and not able to get to the phone in time. Take it with you to the clothesline or when you are outside gardening

meet Edna Edna admitted she had a bad habit of leaving her shoes on the bedroom floor. She had started tripping on them at night when she got up to go to the bathroom. She made a conscious effort to change this habit by re-organising her wardrobe and keeping a special place for her shoes. She said it was hard to do all the time but she rewarded herself last week by going to the pictures because she had gone for one whole week without leaving clutter on the floor.

3. TO MAKE USING THE STAIRS IN MY HOME SAFER:

- ❑ I go down the stairs as quickly as possible.
- ❑ I install a grab rail.
- ❑ I improve the lighting at the top and bottom of the stairs.
- ❑ I install a skylight over the stairs to improve the light during the day.
- ❑ I don't leave the grandchildren's toys on the steps.

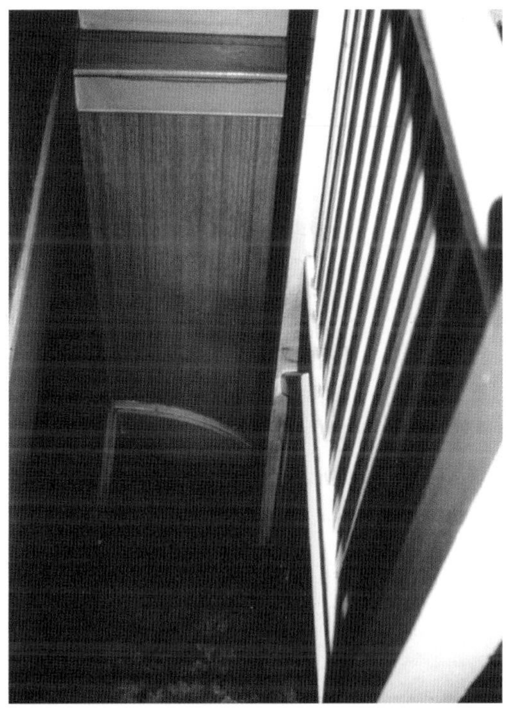

BEFORE: A combination of rushing in loose, slippery-soled shoes and poor visibility could cause a very nasty fall on these steps

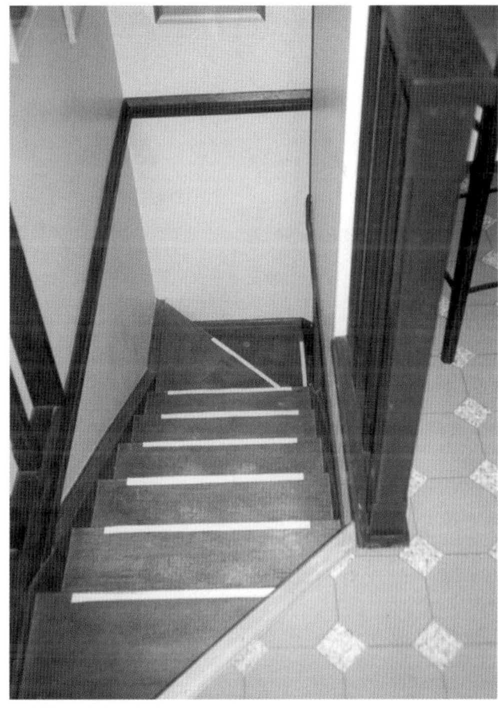

AFTER: The stairs were made safer by lightening their colour, putting in a skylight and putting non-slip strips on the step edges

There are many things you can do to make steps safer. A common hazard point is at the bottom of the steps, where the lighting is often poor and you can just miss the step. Having your vision checked regularly is as important as reviewing the lighting or checking the carpet tread.

4. MY FAVOURITE CHAIR:

❑ Has a soft thick-pile mat in front of the chair to stop the carpet wearing.
❑ Is high enough and has good armrests for standing up easily.
❑ Has a footstool in front of the chair so I can put up my feet.
❑ Is a challenging height for me and reminds me to do my sit-to-stand exercises.

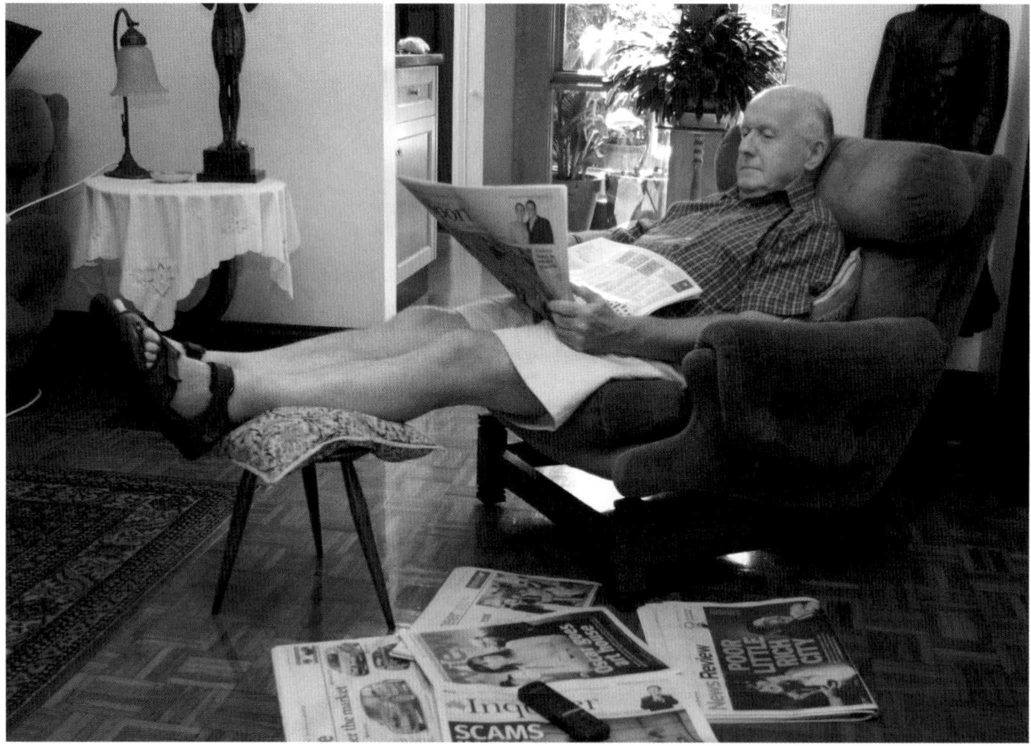

It is hard to decide to remove favourite footstools or mats, particularly as you have placed them there for a reason. But they can be a real hazard and you can easily trip over them when you get up. It's far safer to keep the floor area around your chair clear.

meet Harry Harry was dozing on his comfy lounge chair when the doorbell rang. He jumped up quickly but tripped on his footstool. He is now convinced it's time for a change.

5. TO MAKE THE KITCHEN FLOOR SAFER:

- ❑ I remove all mats.
- ❑ I wipe up spills straightaway.
- ❑ I buy a heavy slip-resistant mat to replace the loose slippery mat at the sink.
- ❑ I always have bare feet so I can feel the slippery patches.

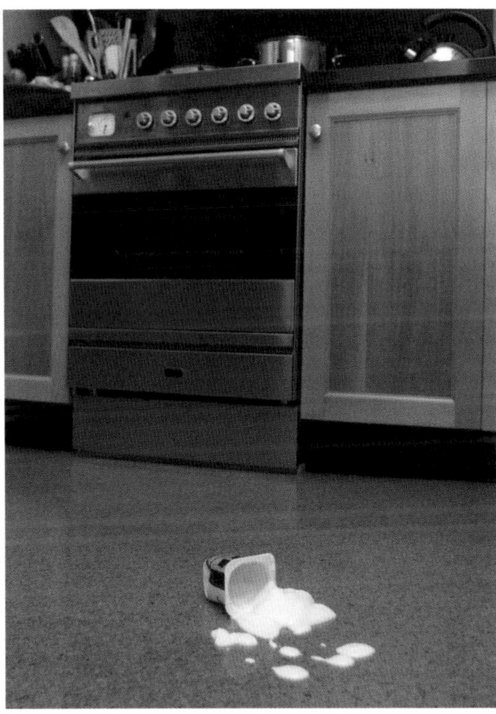

BEFORE: It's easy to slip on a floor when something spills on it

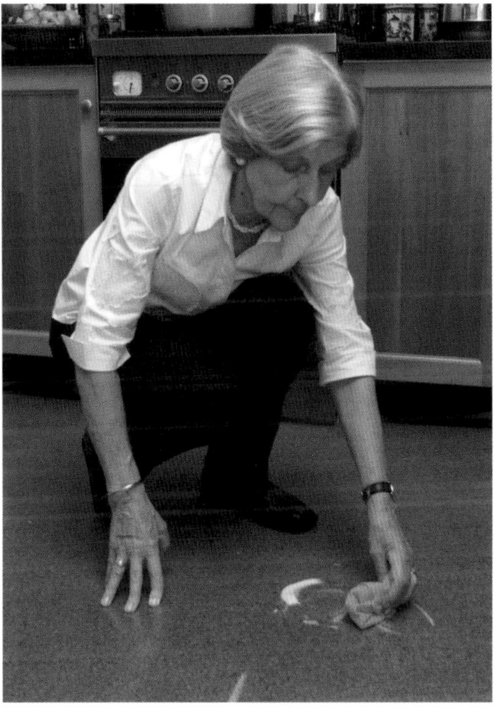

AFTER: As soon as something spills, always wipe it up. That way, you avoid the chance of slipping on the slippery surface

meet Laura Laura works in the restaurant industry. When someone spills something on the restaurant floor, that person shouts "spill" and everyone stays where they are till it's cleaned up. At home she thinks "spill" in her head and this reminds her to clean any spillages up straightaway. If it is oil or butter she always makes sure she uses a bit of detergent to remove the grease.

6. SO THAT I DON'T FALL OVER A CORD ACROSS THE FLOOR:

- ❑ I do not use extension leads.
- ❑ I put tape over the extension lead.
- ❑ I rearrange the furniture so the cord is not across the floor.
- ❑ I use extra leads so they go further.
- ❑ I tape or clip the lead to the walls so that it is not on the floor.

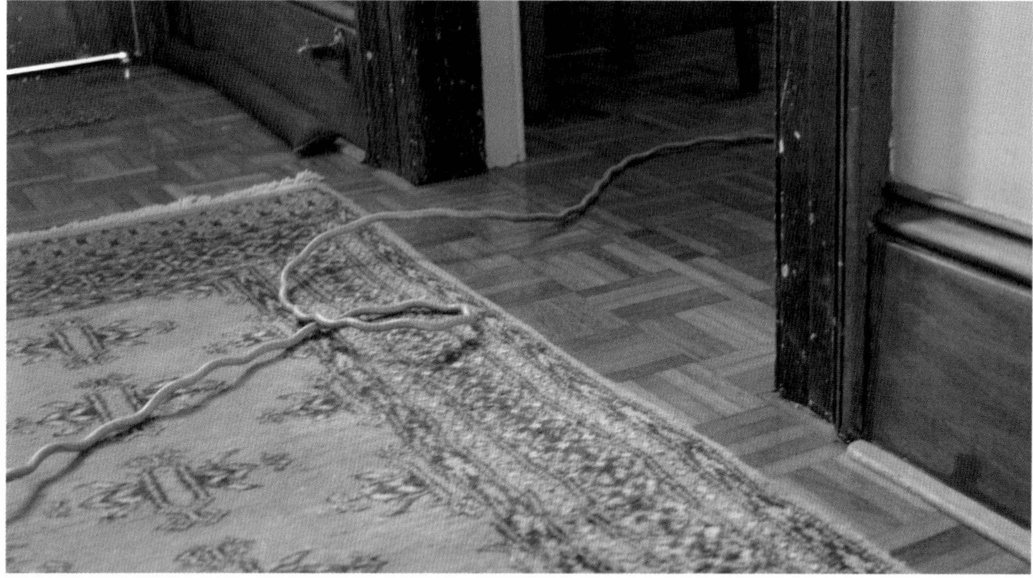

Always keep your walkways free of extension leads and other cords. A clear path means less chance of a fall

meet Alma Alma had severe macular degeneration (this eye condition meant she had very poor vision). Her lead from the electric heater that she uses in winter was the same colour as her carpet, making it nearly impossible to see. It was only by chance that her daughter saw the cord. She realised it could potentially cause Alma to fall, so she got a handyman to secure the heater cord to the skirting board. It is very important to have good heating in winter, particularly as more hip fractures occur on the coldest days, but it is also important to be sure that your set-up is safe.

7. TO CHANGE A LIGHT BULB:

- ❑ I use a step ladder with a firm base and a safety rail to hold on to.
- ❑ I use the kitchen stool to climb on.
- ❑ I put the dining chair on the table and climb up.
- ❑ I ask someone else to do it.

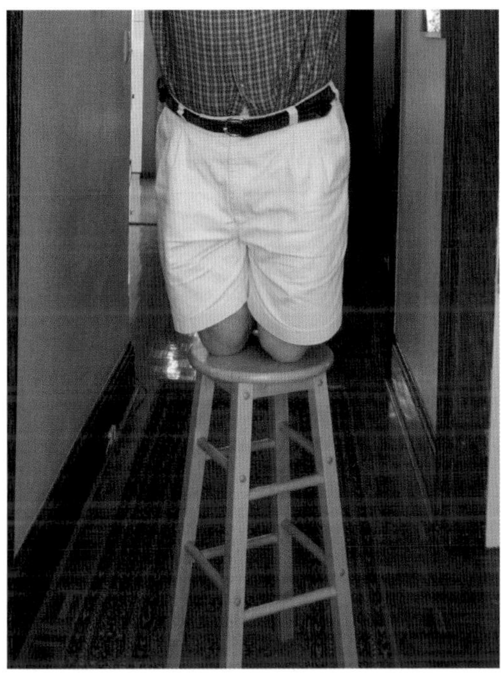

BEFORE: Kneeling on a stool to change a light bulb is dangerous. The stool could topple over and cause a nasty fall

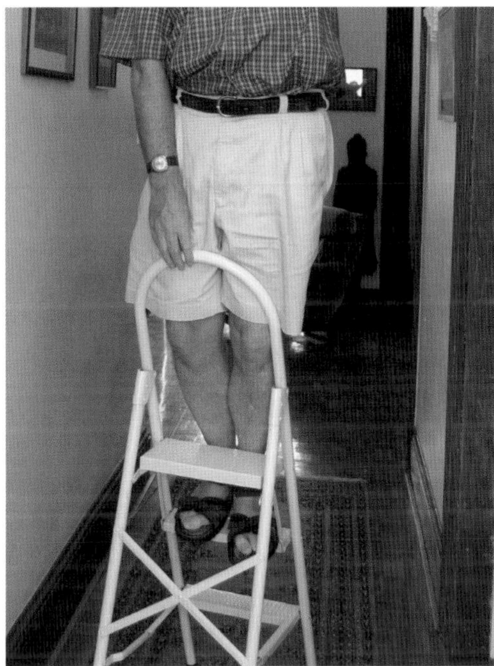

AFTER: Use a step ladder with a firm base and safety rail so you can hold onto the rail with one hand and change the bulb with the other

It's good to know what to look for in a safe step ladder. Safety features include: wide steps, good tread, legs that have rubber grips and being lightweight and foldable so that it easy to put away and get out. When you use the step ladder don't stand on the top rung as you will not be stable enough on it to be truly safe. Plan to store the step ladder in a handy place so you can get to it easily.

8. WHEN I GET UP AT NIGHT:

- ❑ I never switch on a night-light.
- ❑ I have a "touch" lamp beside the bed.
- ❑ I leave a torch beside the bed.
- ❑ I have an LED light plugged in to a power point somewhere along the route to the toilet.

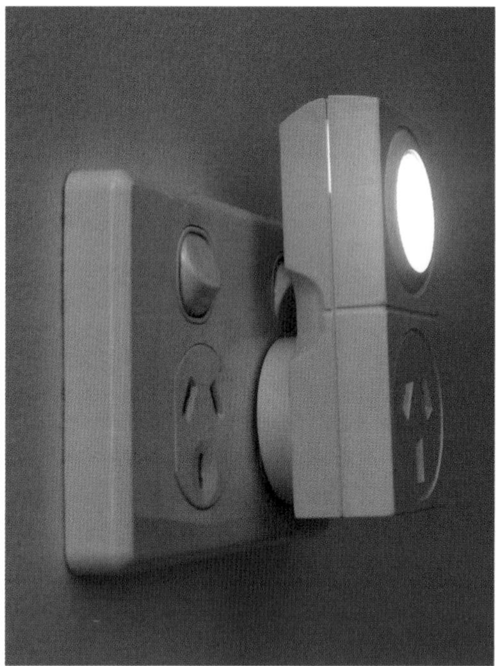

This is what an LED plug-in light looks like. You can buy them in supermarkets and hardware stores

While not as many falls occur at night (probably because people are usually in bed at night), they do still happen. If you don't want to turn on a light, think about the alternatives, such as a LED light that plugs into a power point. This type of light gives an adequate enough glow to make the pathway to the toilet clearly seen.

Safe clothing

Keep your safety in mind when you buy your clothes. Remember that loose-fitting robes and long, free-flowing clothes can catch on doorknobs and furniture. Think about wrapping robes around you snugly and fastening them with a tie or belt instead. Keep hems above the ankle.

You can always make changes so your home environment is safer.

Making changes for safety

You can always make changes so your home environment is safer. For example, if you stick self-adhesive safety strips on step edges, tidy up clutter from traffic ways and stairwells, and improve the lighting for access areas, your home will be safer to move around. And if you take more time to answer the phone, use a step ladder instead of a chair to reach high things or take particular care when you have been unwell or are stressed, your lifestyle will be safer.

meet Shirley

Shirley was looking forward to going to a concert. She had bought a new pair of long pants to wear over her high-heeled shoes. She had a lovely night but when she got home from the concert her feet were killing her so she took off her shoes. She tripped on the long pants while climbing the stairs, and fell flat on her face. When she looked up, her cat was sitting next to her, staring at her as though it was laughing at her vanity.

COMMENT

Shirley would have been better to buy more comfortable shoes or at least to have changed her pants when she took her high heels off.

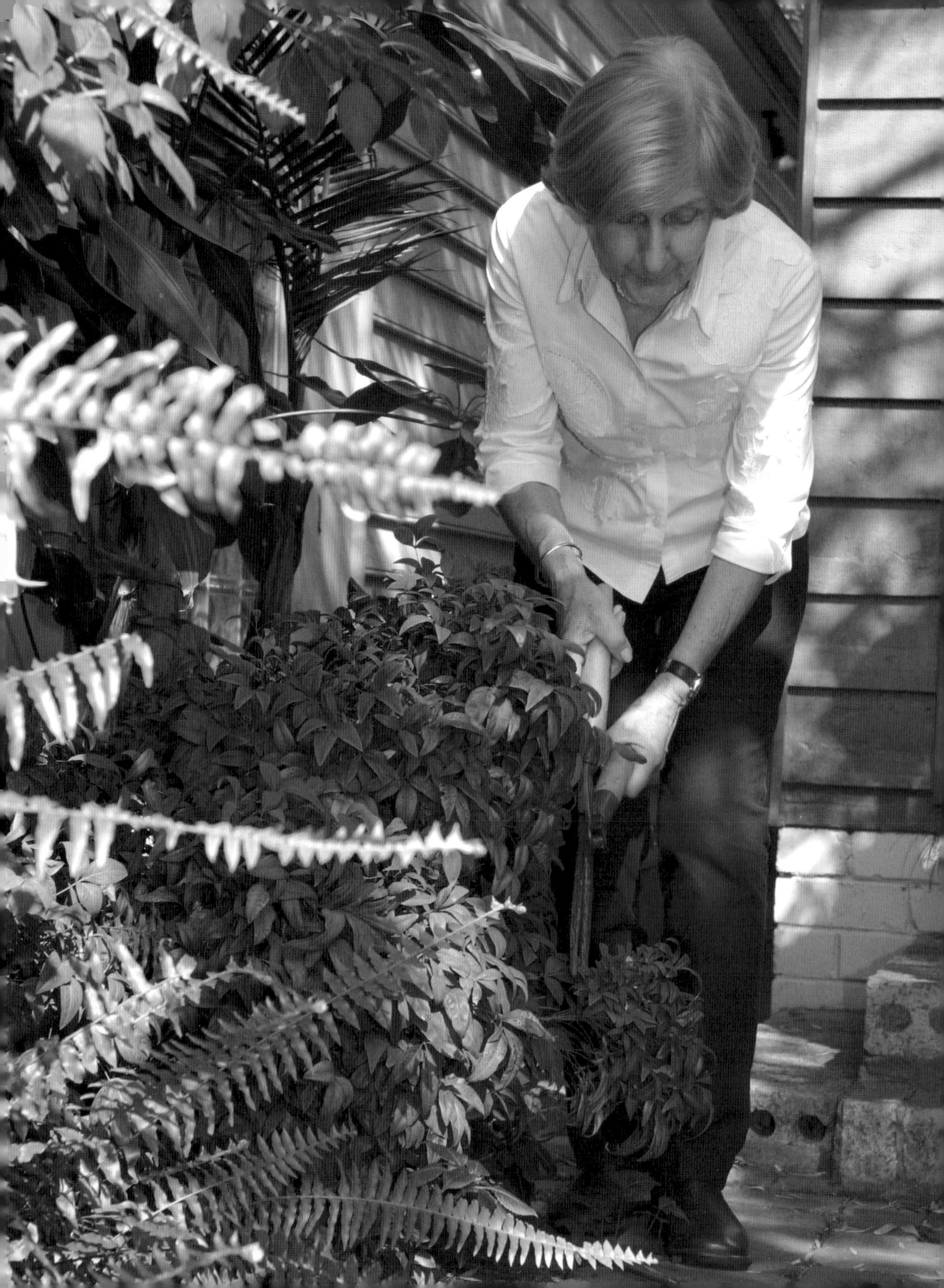

Keeping your pathways clear of overhanging shrubs will reduce your chances of having a fall when you are outside

You may need help to make changes to your home. If you install handrails, remove moss from slippery surfaces, fix uneven pathways, install sensor lights at porches, cut edges to allow more natural light thus preventing build-up of moss, and treat slippery tiles and other surfaces with non-slip products, you will lessen the chances of an accident occurring around your home. To arrange some help, contact your local council or health services and find out if there is a local community scheme. These schemes often provide a low-cost home-handyman service. Ask if they offer the sort of work you require.

Research has shown that if an occupational therapist visits someone at home after they have had a fall, the chance of them falling again is reduced. An occupational therapist can advise you about the hazards in your home. If you want to find out more, contact your local aged-care health service.

Try this

Walk around your home and look for hazards.

- What did you find?
- What could you change about your home environment to remove these hazards?
- What home activities might you do differently now?

CHAPTER 13

community safety

Being able to go out into the community, to meet friends and family, and to do the things you want to do with confidence is the most rewarding part of falls reduction. You'll be able to start achieving this by doing the balance and strength exercises and by developing a good, safe heel–toe walk. However, just like at home, many hazards exist in the wider community.

It's important to become aware of these obstacles and to learn to negotiate them, making behavioural decisions that will ensure your safety.

The strategies in this chapter are closely aligned to the balance and strength exercises from chapters 9 and 10. Increasing your balance and strength coupled with these strategies will help keep you independent and connected to your community.

Assessing your own safety

Have you noticed that you are starting to have difficulty or feel less confident about doing any the following:

- stepping up or down a gutter
- walking up or down a slope
- walking on different surfaces
- walking outside
- shopping
- crossing a road
- walking in a crowd
- catching a bus, train or taxi
- walking around the garden.

If the answer is "yes", it's probably time to introduce ways to improve these activities so that you feel safer and more confident when you are out and about.

Risks in the community

It's important to become aware of these obstacles and to learn to negotiate them, making behavioural decisions that will ensure your safety.

There could be many reasons why you need to pay attention to hazards in the community, especially as you grow older. Your usual pace may be to rush, even though your body might require you to go slower. Your pace may be slower than it used to be, or slowed for a medical reason. It may take longer to cross the road, especially if you often take short cuts and cross the road at a diagonal.

Where you choose to cross the road can impact on your safety, for example, crossing the road in front of parked cars makes you less visible to drivers. Traffic may give you confusing signals, such as, at roundabouts where no two drivers seem to indicate in the same way.

Your decreasing vision may stop you from seeing all the hazards and this may be particularly so in low light conditions. You may not hear traffic, or traffic noise may be confusing.

Kerb ramps and gutters may be getting difficult to negotiate. Uneven pavers and footpaths can be a looming tripping hazard. Slippery areas are also a concern—slippery surfaces such as wet areas, and particularly supermarket floors.

Strategies to enhance your safety when you are on foot:

When you are out and about walking in your local community, keep these strategies in mind:

- take your time. Plan ahead so that you don't need to rush

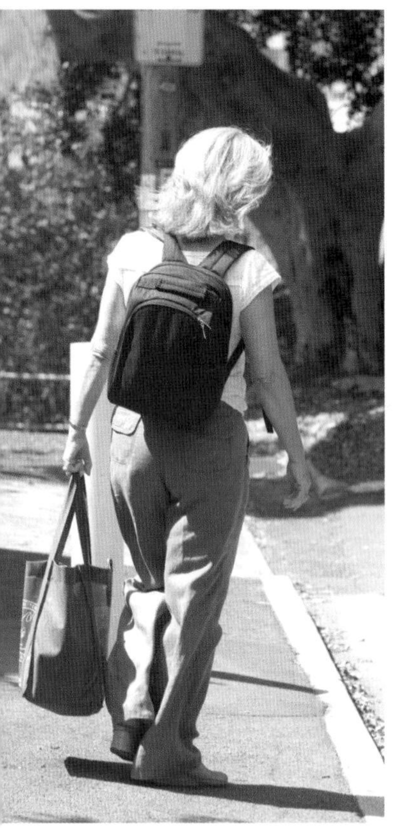

When you want to go out, take your time and plan ahead so that you don't have to rush

- scan a few metres ahead when you walk. As you walk, don't look straight down or too far into the distance. Scanning ahead gives you time to adjust your step and avoid a trip or slip hazard
- walk down kerb ramps or gutters with your feet more apart to give yourself a more stable base
- when stepping up or down at a gutter, pick a spot where there is a pole to hold for support
- wear your glasses and hearing aid when outdoors if you need them
- look around and choose the path with the least number of hazards. The quickest route is not always the safest.

In crowds you can get knocked and jostled. If you are concerned in crowds:

- stop and wait till the crowd moves on
- widen your base of support by moving your feet a little apart to give you a more stable base. This will improve your confidence over areas that are more difficult to negotiate (for example, over grassy terrain or a sloping kerb ramp)
- walk with smaller steps
- strengthen your legs and improve your balance through exercise
- plan your outings for the less busy times, between 10.00 am and 2.00 pm
- use a trolley around the shopping centre
- have your vision checked regularly, though take special care when you first have changes made to your glasses as it could take a while to adjust to your new prescription.

When crossing streets:

- never assume the driver has seen you when you're about to cross the road. Eyeball the driver; even if

you can't see them, look towards the driver. This is a definite communication that you want to cross and they should stop
- cross the road where you can be seen. Walk that extra bit further if necessary to a safe spot. Move away from parked cars and other visual obstructions to motorists
- cross with other people, if possible
- walk to the traffic lights. It is far safer and the exercise is good for you. Remember the flashing red "Don't walk" sign means you can continue your crossing, but you should not start to leave the kerb. The flashing sign is not meant to tell you to rush; it's saying "finish crossing".

People often tell us they get very nervous crossing when the flashing light starts because they feel the light is flashing at them. They have to remind themselves that it is not meant for them but for anyone contemplating leaving the kerb.

Some facts and figures

The green "Walk" sign usually lasts for six seconds and the red flashing "Don't walk" sign lasts longer. It could last up to 15 seconds but the length varies, depending on the width of the road. The formula in NSW is based on 1.2 seconds for every metre; however, the formula used can vary by state and country so it's best to wait for the beginning of a light cycle and give yourself plenty of time to cross.

Avoid crossing at roundabouts. Most drivers seem unsure of the rules that prevail here and cars come from all directions. It is usually much safer to walk further along the road to cross than to try to do so at the roundabout.

If you are going out on dark or cloudy days, at dusk or at night:

- take extra care when it's windy. Walk steadily with your feet further apart where necessary
- wear light-coloured clothing and carry a yellow or light-coloured umbrella
- carry a torch
- put reflective tape around your bag, cane or arm. You can buy this tape from bicycle shops
- hold your bag firmly over your shoulder and walk close to walls to avoid bag snatching.

meet Beryl

Beryl wanted to attend the local handicraft group on Tuesdays and Thursdays. The inner-city suburb where she lived had originally been designed for horses and carts. The gutters were high and the footpaths were uneven, with tree roots lifting pavers along the way. Even though it was a familiar, well-trodden route, she carefully planned the safest and best ways to cross the roads and negotiate where to go. She decided to walk the route in stages, concentrating on walking with a wider-based gait, heel–toe walking and scanning ahead to cope with uneven footpaths.

Scanning ahead made Beryl more prepared for the hazards and gave her time to adjust her step to avoid the hazard. She concentrated on stepping her stronger leg up the gutter first, and she used telegraph poles for support on the most hazardous stretches. She also made sure to wear her sturdiest shoes and cleaned her glasses so she could see well. She went with a friend for the first few times. She shared her goals with her friend and was able to talk them through with her as she went. She found talking about her experience particularly supportive and reinforced her strategies by boosting her confidence.

The following action plan was for Beryl's first two weeks and then she reviewed it. She found that this plan, combined with doing her balance and strength exercises, helped her start to achieve her goal. She now feels much more in touch with other people and feels part of her community again.

Try this

Choose three areas where you are not confident moving about. Draw up an action plan so you focus on getting to know these areas and become confident in them. Pick a long-term goal, such as to walk to the shops, a club or the bus stop. Plan in small steps what you want to practise to achieve this. Plan exactly what you will do, when you will practise it and how often. Practise with a buddy at first until you have enough confidence to go on your own.

	Getting up and down gutters	Walking over uneven pavers and tree roots	Crossing the road
What *exactly* am I going to do?	Use the principle of stronger leg up the gutter first and weaker leg down first. I'll say this out loud to my friend at the first two gutters.	Heel–toe walking and scanning ahead. When I come to a hazard, I'll widen my stance for more support. Walk with a friend.	Avoid the roundabout and walk to the pedestrian crossing. Cross with a friend.
When will I do it?	At each gutter along the route.	Morning practices along the footpath in the block nearest to home.	Between 10.00 am and midday when the roads are less busy.
How often will I do it?	Twice a week when I am going to the centre and returning home.	Every day for three days before trying the walk to the centre.	Three times a week, when I shop and go to the centre.

CHAPTER 14

travel safety

To stay independent in the community, it is as important to have access to good transport as it is to be able to walk safely along the street. Without transport, your range of mobility is severely limited

There are a range of strategies you can use to travel more safely on buses and trains.

But many older people are unable to bear the burden of owning a car and only half the older people living alone in Australia have one. This is largely because of the high costs involved in maintaining a car (up to 30 per cent of total income for people on lower incomes). Studies also show that older people with cars tend to use them less frequently than the average population, and tend to make much shorter trips.

So, public transport is very important to older people. Access to buses, trains and trams facilitates independence and encourages you to be involved in community life at a price within the reach of most people. And yet, for many older people, these benefits are still out of reach. The increased physical risks involved in using bus and train systems can be a major deterrent. In a study conducted in 1998, more than half the participants said that the main reason they did not use public transport was because of the difficulty they had getting into and out of buses or train carriages. Too often, a fear of falling combines with a fear of embarrassment, and people avoid public transport and what it can provide.

Public transport strategies

There are a range of strategies you can use to travel more safely on buses and trains. Of course, our ideas are by no means exhaustive, and many suggestions have come from people who have focused on how to lower their chances of having a fall. We were amazed at the diversity of ideas and experiences that came from the people in our groups and it was always pleasing to hear how they found new confidence by taking more control, planning ahead and getting results.

Special access

Some buses and trains have special access facilities for older people. The buses allow easy access on and off the bus and are not just for wheelchair access. The accessible buses are lower to the ground, have a "kneeling" action that lowers them for easier entry, and space up front for wheelchairs or larger walking aids. See pages 158–9 for details of what's on offer in your state.

meet Juliette

Juliette noticed that, lately people had been offering her a seat on the bus. She wondered why they were doing this but acknowledged that it must have been because of her white hair. At first she was resistant to the idea, but now she's grateful for the offers as she realises her limitations and knows she's more stable when she's sitting down. Juliette always wears a small backpack now to keep both her hands free. At first she thought some of the tips for community safety were very basic and just commonsense. However, she says it has been very worthwhile reminding herself to do things like not getting up until the bus stops and having her money out before she gets on the bus.

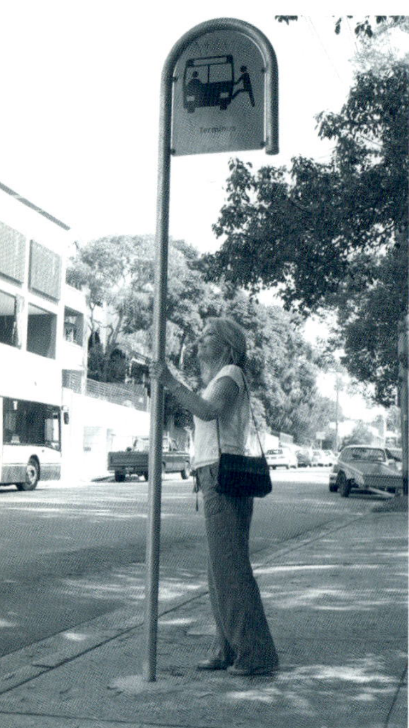

Be at the bus stop early so you can be the first to get onto the bus

Strategies for safe bus travel

Before you get on the bus:

- have your money ready
- be early at the bus stop so you can get on first
- try to travel in non-peak times (10 am to 2 pm) when there are fewer people to contend with
- take a backpack in case you see things to buy. A small lightweight backpack leaves your hands free to hold on to things in the bus and keeps you steady. As an alternative, an "over the opposite shoulder" bag is less intrusive than a backpack, but still leaves the hands free
- plan to go to the bigger shops with a friend on a bus trip
- find out which buses in your state have access facilities and how they are indicated. See pages 158–9 for contact details.

On the bus:

- ask the driver not to take off until you're seated
- take the first seat, up front if possible
- keep a hand free to hold onto a seat or pole
- don't get out of your seat or change seats while the bus is moving. If you are moving about the bus while it is in motion, it is far more likely that you will slip and hurt yourself, not to mention bump into the other passengers.

Getting off the bus:

- always ask the bus driver to pull up as close to the gutter as possible
- when you get off the bus, pause, then walk in the same direction the bus is travelling in, at least until you feel steady and confident. Shirley, a retired bus conductor, gave us this somewhat

Once you are off the bus, hold on to a pole to support you as you step up the gutter

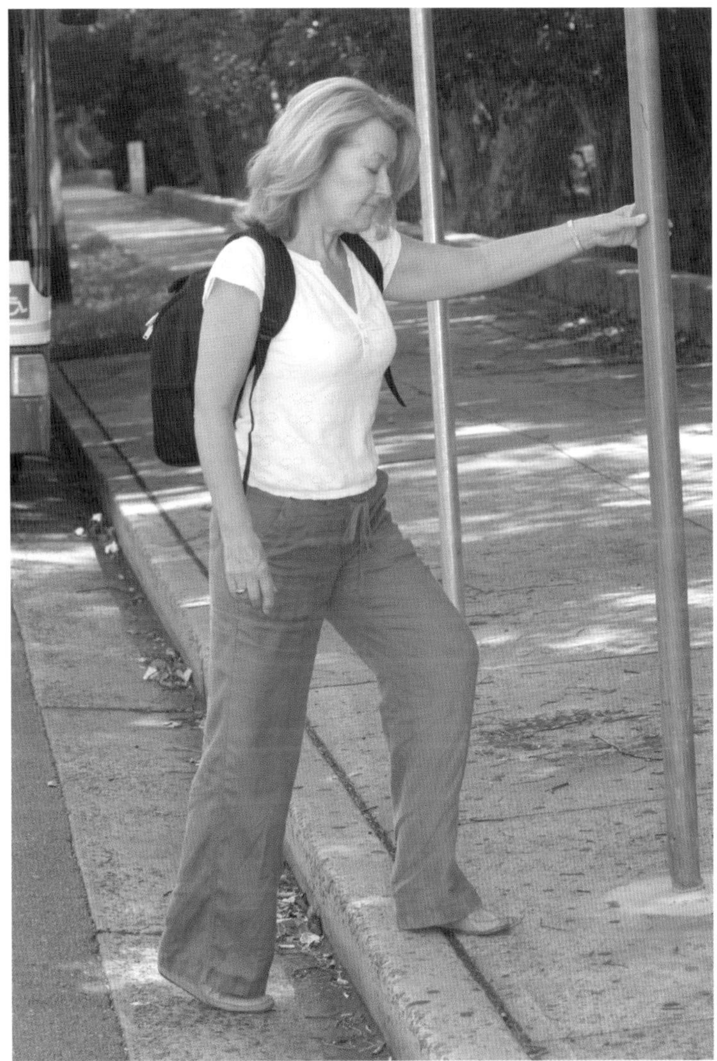

curious tip. She had worked on the buses for over forty years. She said she would often suggest this tip to someone who looked a little unsteady when getting off the bus

- if you have trouble with your knees, go down the bus steps sideways, or even backwards
- hang on to the pole for the bus stop sign to help you step up the gutter

Right: Hold onto the bus's handrail for support as you step on to the bus

Responding to needs

People in the community are generally getting more assertive, and both government and private bus providers are recognising the diverse needs of mature travellers. In the five years since we have been running our Stepping On programs, we have observed that people are feeling more able to tell bus drivers what they need. In return, the drivers are responding.

Transport providers are also investing time and effort in making travel more accessible for everyone. Initiatives include providing information on timetables about easy-access buses so you can plan your journey ahead, and playing recorded information, such as which train stations have lifts and ramps, at booking offices to make communication easier. This information can be available by contacting your local rail or bus service.

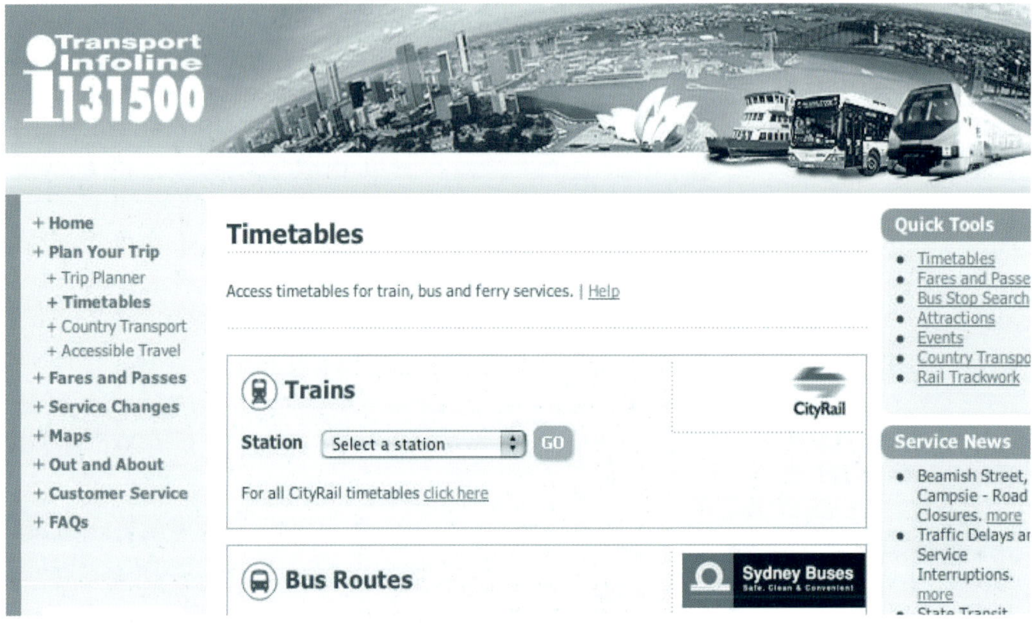

You can look up the timetables for buses, trains, trams and ferries on the Internet

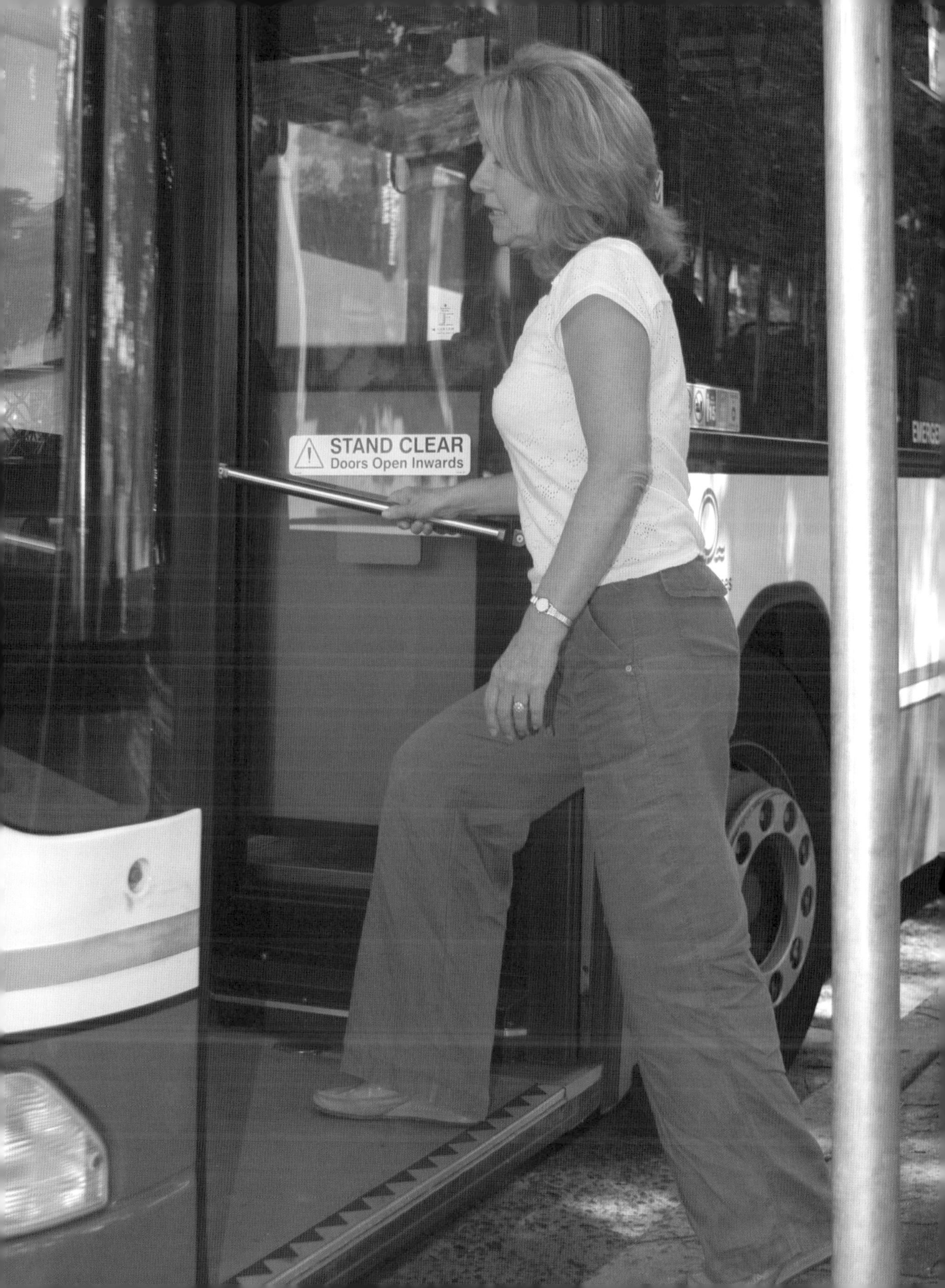
STAND CLEAR
Doors Open Inwards

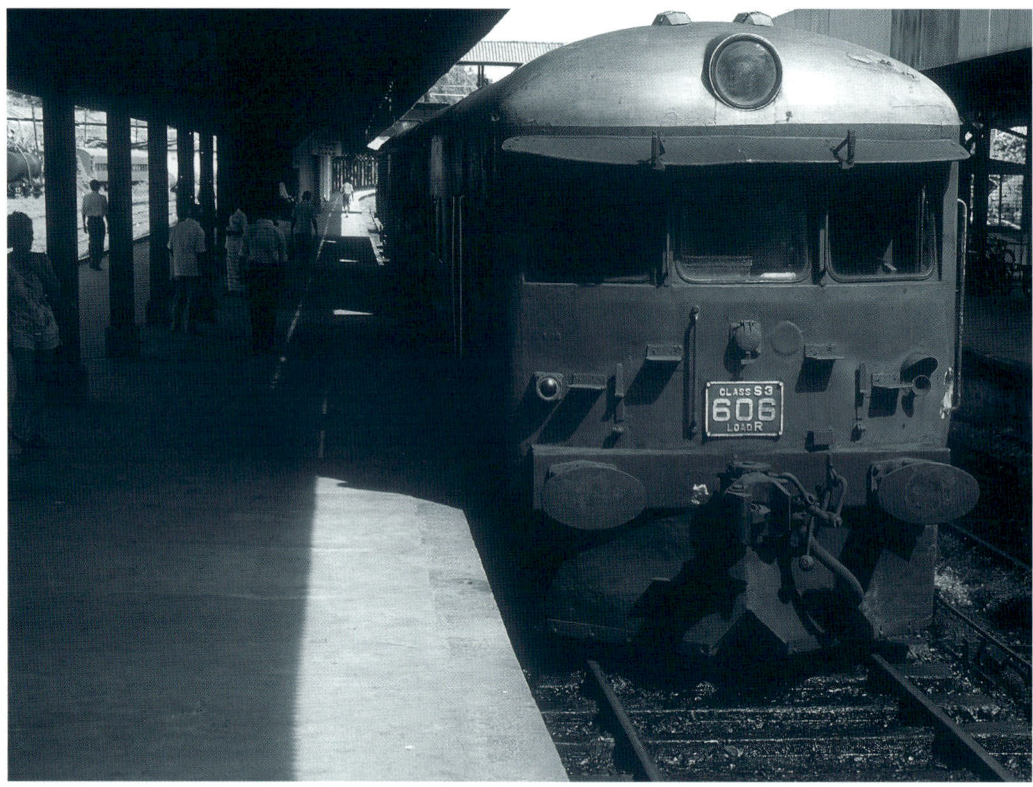

You can always call your local train station to find out where and when the train gets to your station

Strategies for safe train travel

Before you get on the train:

- be early at the station so you don't have to rush
- ask the ticket seller which platform you catch your train from
- ring ahead to find out about the station you are leaving from or travelling to. Find out whether it has a lift and whether the steps have a handrail
- if you use a walking stick, take it with you
- travel in non-peak times (10 am to 2 pm) when there are fewer people around
- if you have a disability, ring the destination station before you travel and ask for extra help getting off when you arrive.

If you have trouble with your knees, try getting off the train sideways, holding the pole near the door for support.

Getting on and off the train:

- if you have luggage, ask the guard (or someone on the station or train) to help you with it
- take your time getting on or off. The train guard will not allow the train to move while you are getting on or off
- some states have a guard's carriage. This is often in the middle of the platform and in some states has a blue light above the door or a blue compartment door
- sit in the ground-level area to avoid the stairs
- if you have trouble with your knees, try getting off the train sideways, holding the pole near the door for support.

Local knowledge

It's a good idea to get to know the train transport in your own area so that you can use it safely. Keep a chart with details on the stations you use regularly. Include information on:

- stairs have a handrail (yes/no)
- ticket office broadcasts information about access (yes/no)
- taxis and buses are nearby (yes/no)
- station has a lift (yes/no)
- station has an escalator (yes/no)

Some train stations are designated easy-access stations. See pages 158–9 for details in your state.

CHAPTER 15

footwear

Shoes are fun to choose and good to wear. Popular opinion says that women just love to buy shoes, and men tend to stick to their favourites. In some ways, our shoes reflect who we are.

The shoe choices we make are a part of how we express ourselves. But choosing safe, sensible shoes is important in maintaining your balance and stability as you move about.

Shoes are personal. People buy them for comfort and appearance but safety is rarely a high priority. Many falls at home occur when people are wearing shoes that are not firmly fastened or are loose-fitting. Many people wear slippers when they are at home but worn-out slippers will cause you to shuffle because they do not encourage heel–toe walking. You may not have noticed that the soles of your heels have become worn. What was once a safe pair of shoes may no longer give support because the heels are uneven and slippery.

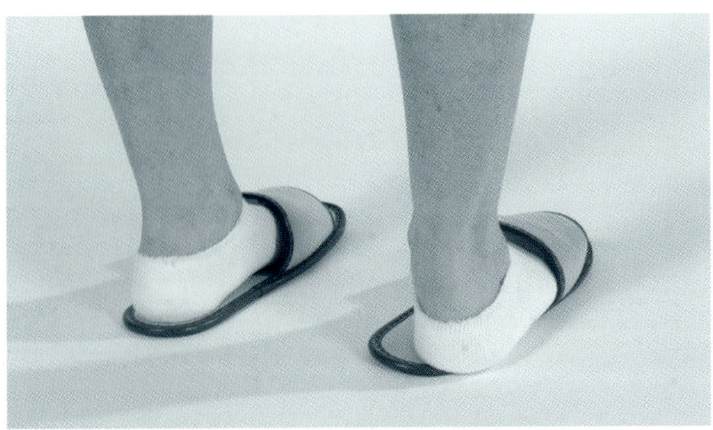

Never wear slip-on scuffs. They don't give your feet any support and you can trip in them too easily

In some ways, our shoes reflect who we are.

Features of safe shoes: the "four safety features" audit

When buying safe shoes, remember that price does not always indicate safeness. There are four main features you should look out for when buying safe shoes.

SHOES NEED TO:

- give good support
- fit your feet well
- have a sole that grips
- have a heel that provides stability and grip.

A SUPPORTIVE SHOE

Your shoes should have secure fastenings. They need a firm arch to support the arch of your foot and to offer stability. They should cover most of your foot and provide a firm and snug fit for your heel.

A GOOD FIT

Your shoe should hold the foot well back into the shoe so that your heel rests neatly in the heel of the shoe and you don't flop forwards. It also needs to have a roomy toe area so that your toes feel comfortable and not cramped. Allow at least 1.2 centimetres between your longest toe and the end of the shoe. Have your feet measured properly by a shoe specialist so that your shoes will fit correctly.

A SOLE THAT GRIPS

Your shoes need a non-slip rubber sole that is textured for grip. Turn your shoe over and look at the sole. Is it shiny and worn? If so, the shoe may need to be resoled, or if unrepairable, thrown away and replaced. Don't forget to check the sole of any new shoes you are considering to buy.

A STABLE HEEL THAT GRIPS

Most slips and falls from bad footwear happen when the back of your heel strikes the ground. The heel needs to have a textured surface for traction, with a pattern and depth that will penetrate any spills or lubricant on the floor and will grip less resistant surfaces.

A low and broad heel is best for stability and safe walking. But if you have been used to wearing high heels, you should not suddenly wear flat shoes as your tendons may need time to stretch. You'll need to adapt gradually to a lower heel.

Be wary of smooth-soled shoes, particularly leather-soled styles.

TRY THIS

You can give new shoes with shiny leather soles some traction by "scoring" the soles—rub them on concrete before you wear them. There are also commercial rubber solutions that you can paint on to the soles of your shoes to prevent them from being slippery. Ask at your hardware store or shoe repairer.

Looking after your feet

Researchers into falls are only just beginning to unravel the risks associated with the physiology of the foot. It seems that foot pain, and big toe and foot joint deformities, are associated with falls risk. So if you suffer from any foot pain or any foot deformity, take particular care with your feet and footwear choices. Well-fitting and supportive footwear with sufficient toe room should always be worn.

Foot care is recommended to keep your falls risk down. Reducing or removing calluses as well as general education about foot care is beneficial. Regular visits to or home visits by a podiatrist provide good management of this. If your foot tends to roll inwards or roll outwards, then orthotics will help you grip the ground with more stability and assist you with a normal heel–toe stride. Your podiatrist can give you a referral for orthotic shoe inserts to realign your step if required.

Footwear check list

- make a personal list of the pros and cons of wearing safer shoes
- think about the four audit features to check out your shoes and slippers: stability, fit, sole and heel. Fix the problems if you can; otherwise, replace your dangerous footwear with safer styles
- use the four audit features to guide you in buying some safer shoes that you like the look of and that are comfortable

meet Beatrice Beatrice was visiting her daughter while recovering from a urinary tract infection. She brought her favourite slippers with her. They were big, fluffy dog slippers with a tartan hat and a tongue hanging out. She had had them for years, a gift from the grandchildren. The slippers gave her no support; they were a very loose fit and made her shuffle; the soles had worn down to a glossy sheen. One night, as she got out of bed and walked across the polished wooden floor in the slippers, she fell, breaking her hip. Beatrice explained how difficult it was to be sensible instead of sentimental when considering her slippers and how now, with hindsight, she sees things differently.

CHAPTER 16

hip protection

Hip protectors are special hip shields that protect you from fracturing your hip if you fall.

Bruce said that hip protectors were like the "box" in cricket or "cup" in American football, just worn in a different place!

Hip protector inserts are small plastic shields that slip into pockets in specially designed underwear, worn over the top of your usual underwear. They are designed so that they sit firmly over the hip and do not slip away on impact. Some people have been a bit reluctant to wear them but they are quite comfortable, lightweight, and barely visible through your clothes. If they are worn correctly, they are very effective in reducing the effect of a fall on your hip. It is rare to break your hip if you fall while wearing one.

Hip protectors are designed to absorb the impact and redistribute the forces from the hip to the thigh muscles. They are similar to protective gear that is worn in many sports. In one of our groups, Bruce commented that they were like the "box" in cricket or "cup" in American football, just worn in a different place!

Hip protectors not only help prevent hip fractures but they give you a great sense of security. They are a very good option for people who have previously restricted their activity because they have a fear of falling. Wearing the protectors also boosts your confidence in situations of change, such as returning to bowls after a fall or visiting a relative overseas and worrying about being a burden.

To find out more, contact your local health centre or aged services team or look on the Internet for

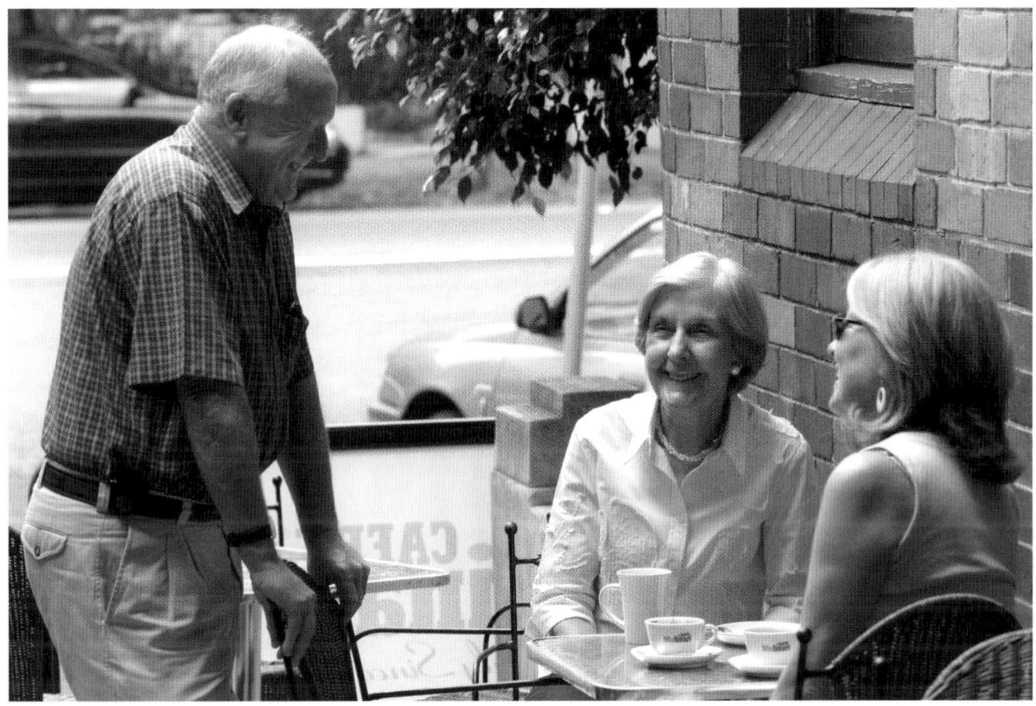

meet Margaret Margaret was shopping in the city. The historic building she was in had just been renovated using glazed tiles, and it had been raining. Margaret turned too quickly and fell hard on her side in the open area. She felt embarrassed and helpless. A lady helped her up and they sat together on the ornate spiral staircase while Margaret composed herself. The helper told Margaret about the hip protectors she wore and let her feel her hips to show she was actually wearing them. She explained how wearing the protectors gave her the confidence to go out, doing all the things she wanted to do in her busy day. Hearing that, Margaret decided to get some herself.

"hip savers" or "hip protectors". The specialised underwear choices for women are improving all the time with a choice of colour and fabric now available. There is also underwear now available for men and also for those with incontinence.

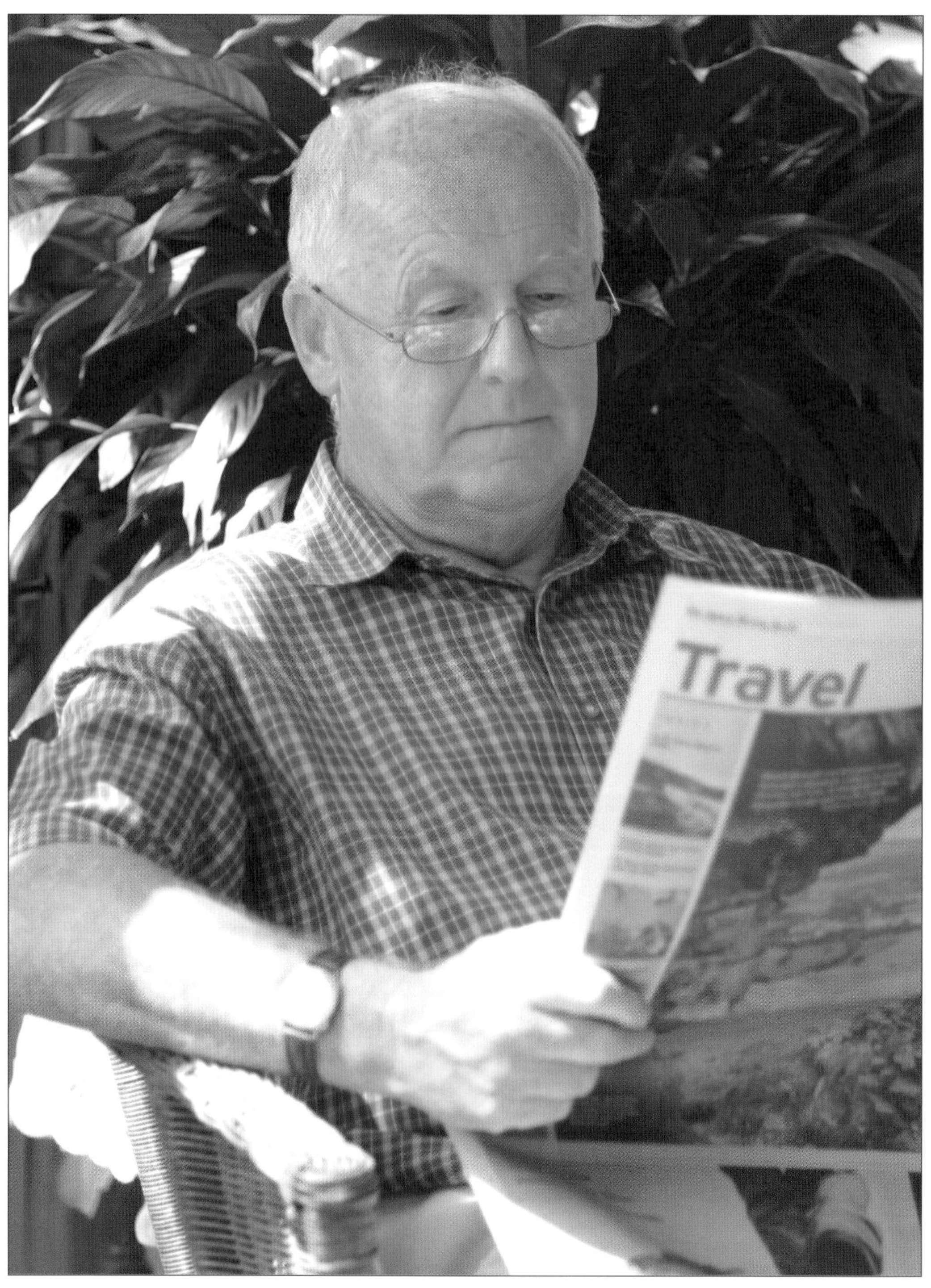
Travel

how to handle a changing body

CHAPTER 17
changing vision

Many studies have shown that poor vision greatly increases the chances of having a fall. In many ways, this is just commonsense. If you have trouble seeing the path ahead, you are liable to misjudge a hazard or even be completely unaware of it until it is too late.

Decreased vision and certain eye diseases are associated with the ageing process. Cataracts can make it difficult to see when moving about and research shows a strong link between cataracts and falls. So it seems fading vision is a clear sign that getting older is directly linked to having more falls. That said, it is not a direct relationship. There is a lot you can do to improve the age–falls relationship as your eyesight becomes less sharp. The main recommendations are:

- have regular eye checks
- get a referral promptly for cataract treatment
- use strategies to cope with low vision.

Statistics show that about half of all people with impaired vision could correct their vision problem by getting new glasses. Furthermore, people with cataracts considerably reduce their chances of fracturing a bone from a fall by having their cataracts treated early. This really is good news. It means that if you correct the hazy vision caused by cataracts, you will reduce your chances of a hip fracture. So if you think you could have cataracts, don't delay. Talk to your doctor and have them treated as soon as possible.

If you can't fix your poor vision, there are strategies to help you see better with the level

"I had no idea that my eyesight and falling over were related. It was in the dark and I completely lost my balance. I felt like I was drunk!"

BESSIE

of vision you have, such as improving the lighting around your home or making sure the edges of steps are clearly defined.

Poor vision can cause problems in all kinds of conditions. The most common problems generally involve misjudging or not seeing clearly the edges of gutters, paths and other obstacles in your path of travel. These can occur with most eyesight problems. Other problems stem from having an intolerance to poor lighting, adjusting from light to dark areas or coping with glare.

The range of visual difficulties

The following eyesight problems are common. Do you know if you have any of these conditions? You may have one of them but it has not been diagnosed. An eye check-up will reveal any of these conditions.

- **CONTRAST SENSITIVITY** Losing the ability to easily see the contrast between light and dark, which thus creates difficulty seeing the edges of borders, obstructions and clutter.
- **LOSS OF A FIELD OF VISION** Loss of central vision in conditions such as macular degeneration and the tunnel vision associated with untreated glaucoma. Tunnel vision is the reverse of losing your central vision. In tunnel vision you lose the vision around the periphery of your sight—it's like looking into a tunnel wherever you gaze. Glaucoma is treatable if picked up early enough, so have your eyes checked regularly for this condition.
- **REDUCED DEPTH PERCEPTION** Difficulty perceiving the relative distance and position of objects, often produced from poor vision in one eye.
- **IMPAIRED DARK ADAPTATION** Difficulty adapting to low-light conditions, especially at night or when

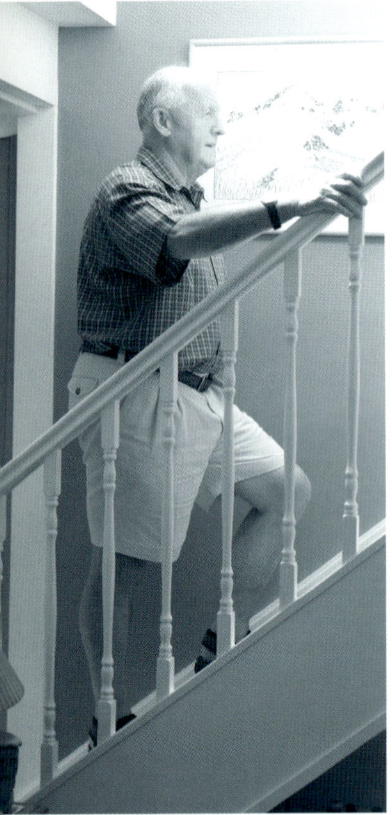

Think about installing a fluorescent light or even a skylight to give good light on your stairs

moving from light to very dark conditions. When this happens, you can feel a bit disoriented and your balance might become unstable.

- **REDUCED COLOUR PERCEPTION** A broad term for difficulty distinguishing between certain colours, also known as "colour blindness". It can reduce your ability to notice obstacles or see steps or other changes in levels.

How to see better and fall less

The simplest and most effective way to reduce the risk of vision-related falls is to have your eyes checked every two years by an eye doctor or optometrist. You tend to get used to your slowly declining vision and learn to live with it. Your eye doctor can pick up any eye diseases, glaucoma for example, and will assess your eyes for the best prescription for glasses.

If you do not already see an optometrist, find one in your local directory or ask your doctor for a referral, then make an appointment. This is one of the most powerful messages to come out of recent research into the visual causes of falling. When you first get new glasses, however, you need to take care while you get used to the new lens changes.

Bifocals and multifocals

Bifocal glasses are great for seeing long and short distances at the same time. However, they can make the edges of steps, paving, gutters and stairs difficult to see. It is easy to misjudge, forget or get confused about which part of the lens to use, so you need to be wary of bifocals and learn to adjust your head to look through the right part of the lens for the right circumstances. If you don't need to wear bifocals to climb the stairs, take them off to avoid any risk.

Lighting

Enhance the light in dimly lit areas and around hazards such as stairs and edges.

It's good to increase the wattage of light bulbs at home, especially if your eyes have difficulty adapting to dark to light changes or have contrast sensitivity. If you currently use low-wattage globes, upgrade to 75- or 100-watt globes. Think about particularly enhancing the light in dimly lit areas and around hazards such as stairs and edges. This will increase visual clarity and help you to detect contrasts and edges. Increased wattage does use more energy, but the increase to your electricity bill will be barely noticeable, and you will be safer.

If your vision is very poor, it's best to have an electrician install broad-spectrum fluorescent lighting. This will give off a more natural type of light, often preferred by older people. Compact fluorescent light bulbs last around eight times longer than normal bulbs and use up to 80 per cent less energy. The highest quality fluorescent tubes are called triphosphorous. They emit a broader spectrum of light and give off the most natural light.

Make the most of natural light in the home. This may involve structural changes such as installing a skylight, or simply opening the curtains. Light-coloured walls and furnishings will also enhance illumination, although be sure to maintain some colour contrast between floor coverings and furniture.

Consider lighting variations at different times, in different seasons and in specific areas such as doorways, step landings and routes to the bathroom. Think about moving any furniture that casts shadows. If glare is a problem, check for reflective surfaces and

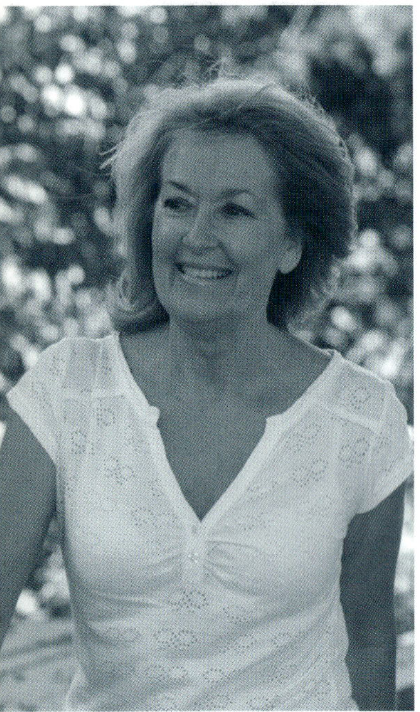

When you've been out, give your eyes a moment to adjust to the different light inside

unshielded light bulbs and work out how you can remove them or rearrange them in the room.

Changes at home

- clutter can make it more difficult to see hazards in your way. Make sure that your hallway, porch and verandah are clear of unnecessary items. Don't use thoroughfares as storage areas
- get rid of furniture with casters or wide legs that may intrude into traffic ways where you walk. The bit that sticks out is easy to trip over. The "sausages" used to stop drafts under doors are a big hazard; it's best to remove them
- make sure there is enough colour contrast between your furniture and walls, curtains and floorings. Consider changing the colour of your furniture or furnishings so that there is enough contrast to make your furniture easy to see. For example, it can be momentarily hard to see a light-coloured coffee table on a light carpet but you can see a dark coffee table on a light carpet out of the corner of your eye
- use safety strips of a contrasting colour to highlight the edges of steps or stairs. Falls on steps often occur because you misjudge the bottom step

Other simple ideas

- when you come inside after being out, wait for a moment before moving about while your eyes adjust to the new light. Your eyes often need a few seconds to catch up with the change in light levels
- when you are outdoors, scan ahead for hazards and if you see one, allow time to adjust your gait

When you are outdoors, scan ahead for hazards.

and avoid the danger spot. Scan ahead as far as you can see—about four to six steps (or equal to a car length) is ideal—but the distance will depend on your vision and how well you can adjust your step to avoid the hazard. And remember you usually need to look down on reaching the hazard in order to negotiate it safely

- be careful of pets—they're easy to trip over! Feed them away from access points and traffic ways
- if you spill something, wipe it up straightaway
- remove slippery moss from pathways as soon as you notice it forming.

Try this

- make an appointment to get your eyes tested
- stand back and observe the lighting in your home. Can you improve it? Would higher-wattage globes work or do you need to think about fluorescent lighting? Do the entrances of your home need some additional lighting?

meet Bill Bill had severe glaucoma that had been untreated so his eyesight was poor. After doing the balance and strength exercises for a few weeks, he wanted to get even fitter, but his wife had osteoarthritis and could not partner him on his walks. Bill's doctor suggested he get a treadmill. Instead, we linked him up with the orientation and mobility instructor from the Low Vision clinic (see page 159). The instructor accompanied him on several walks around the block, giving him suggestions about scanning and defensive walking techniques that would allow for his vision impairment. She helped him become familiar with his local area and to gain confidence. He now enjoys going for his daily walk and feels part of the community.

CHAPTER 18

managing medication

Drugs exist for a good reason. They are designed to help your body get better and stay well so that you can get on with your life. But problems with drugs can arise when you start to take more than one medication. People who take a mix of medications are at a much higher risk of falling.

Some specific and commonly prescribed drugs are known to increase the risk of falls.

This is because drugs can have conflicting effects, reacting with each other to provoke side effects such as dizziness, drowsiness, a dampening of sensation and so on. Many drugs can cause negative side effects on their own, especially if not taken in the appropriate way or if your body is naturally allergic to them. But if you combine incompatible drugs, the negative side effects are likely to be more frequent and more intense.

Some specific and commonly prescribed drugs are known to increase the risk of falls. Sleeping tablets as well as drugs for anxiety or depression have all been proven to significantly increase a person's risk of falls. These drugs can reduce your attentiveness to your surroundings, slow your movements and impair your balance.

If you are on these medications, you may be able to reduce your dosage to safer levels; it is worth discussing this with your doctor. We strongly recommend that you look into the underlying causes of your sleep problems and/or find alternative remedies rather than taking these types of drugs, especially sleeping tablets, for a long time. Alternatives to sleeping tablets are discussed later in this chapter.

Managing multiple medications

To avoid any unnecessary negative side effects as you grow older, have your doctor review your medications and dosages on a regular basis. Your doctor may not be aware of what medication a specialist has given you, or they may not recall all the medications they have prescribed for you in the past. So a review is a good way to reveal all this. Surprisingly, this process does not have a set routine; you usually have to initiate it yourself. Essentially, you need to "take stock" of all the medications you are taking at the moment. Make a list of them and think of any questions you would like answered. Then go to your doctor or pharmacist and use their

meet Daisy

Daisy was going on a bus trip to Wagga. She arranged for someone to look after the cat, water the plants and collect the mail. Before she left, she went to the doctor to get a repeat prescription for her blood pressure tablets. The doctor reviewed her medication and changed the tablets. She had not been on a bus trip for many years and was very excited. That morning she started taking her new medication. As Daisy got off the bus at the lunch stopover, she felt dizzy walking down the steps and fell, fracturing her shoulder.

COMMENT

Daisy's dizziness may have been a side effect of the new drug. Changing medication at the same time as going on a busy holiday is not such a good idea. Daisy was taking numerous other medications and their combination could have resulted in dizziness. She may not have asked enough questions of her doctor or pharmacist about the new medication. Daisy may not have understood when and how to take the dosage.

expert knowledge to make sure you are taking the right medication at the right dosages, and that there are no adverse interactions between them.

Preparing your medication record

You can get a Medicine Record Card from pharmaceutical societies, other organisations and some pharmacies—or make up your own list of medications and dosages by copying the one on page 159. Include all alternative medicines and remedies in your list as these can sometimes interact adversely with other drugs. It is in exactly these situations that a medication review can help sort out what you should take. Your sample headings could be:

- date prescribed
- medicine name
- what it is for
- dose and how often (for example, 2 tablets, three times a day)
- special instructions/warnings (for example, take one hour before a meal)/time of day for dosage (for example, before breakfast)

Two-way information

When you go to your doctor or pharmacist, you are being offered a well-qualified service. But the communication must be two-way. You have the right to know what drugs are going into your body and why, and you will need to be assertive to make sure you find out. It often helps to make a detailed list of the things you would like to know from your doctor or pharmacist and questions you would like to ask, so that everything is covered. If you cannot get

You have the right to know what drugs are going into your body and why, and you will need to be assertive to make sure you find out.

through it all in one session, book another appointment, perhaps even a longer consultation. Here are some examples of questions to ask your doctor and/or pharmacist about your medicines:

- What is the medicine for?
- What does it do? What results can I expect?
- Will this medicine interact with others I am taking?
- How and when do I take it?
- What can I do to lessen the side effects? Are there any things I need to avoid?
- How long do I need to take it? When should it be stopped, or reviewed?
- The bottle can be hard to open; can I get the same tablets in a blister pack?

Knowing what you are taking

While the doctor and pharmacist are responsible for supplying your medication, it is your own responsibility to take reasonable care to reduce the known side effects. Here are some tips to help you adopt this responsibility:

- avoid sleeping tablets in the longer term. They are addictive. Try alternatives—remember a prescription for a night can turn into a prescription for life

meet George George wrote all his medications down on a card, including his hay fever tablets, and took the card to his doctor. The doctor was shocked. "My goodness! How many tablets are you taking?" she said. "I'll have to book you in for a 45-minute consultation to go through each one of these. A standard 15-minute session is not long enough." George came back the next week for a longer session and went through everything with his doctor. As a result, his medications have been halved and he feels much better.

- review dosages of anxiety tablets regularly with your doctor as their side effects can cause falls
- know when, how, and how much medication to take—and stick to it. A dosage dispenser aid may be useful if you have several medications. This is a box that carries your medication and is divided into compartments for each day of the week. It allows you to set out your dosages a week in advance so that you are less likely to forget something or to make a mistake
- start taking a new drug or a higher dosage when you know you are not going to be busy, perhaps on the weekend. If you live alone, take it when you know someone is likely to be around
- don't take someone else's medication. It might have a very different effect on your body
- plan for your holidays in advance. We all tend to race around and do all those things we've been meaning to do for a while at the last minute. Don't leave it till the last minute to change your medication or get a new drug. Give yourself time to adjust to the changes to your body well before you leave for your holiday

meet Steven Steven had mentioned to his doctor that he was taking ten separate tablets and he was worried about their effects. The doctor told him that he was eligible for a government-funded program where a pharmacist would visit Steven's house for an hour to review his medications. So Steven arranged this. The pharmacist helped him to sort out when and how many medications he needed to take. He quickly realised he'd been taking too much. He also understood better why he was taking them, and the possible side effects of the mix he was on. It made him feel better and more in control .

- take special care if you are aware that dizziness is a side effect of any medication. When you get up out of bed, move slowly. Pause before you get up and again before you walk off. This is also a useful strategy for getting out of a chair or a car or for getting off the bus.

Because your pharmacist knows a lot about your medication and dispenses it to you, they are the most important person to help you manage your medications safely.

Get to know your pharmacist

It's a good idea to get to know a local pharmacist. Many pharmacists will offer their time to help you understand side effects and how to take your medications safely. They will be happy to get to know you and your needs. Because your pharmacist knows a lot about your medication and dispenses it to you, they are the most important person to help you manage your medications safely.

Your pharmacist can make up a medication blister pack on a weekly basis. The blister pack is set out in a daily schedule, with each day's tablets contained in one "blister". You push out your daily tablets from each blister. People who have difficulty managing the blister can get a small cutting tool which opens each blister neatly into a cup.

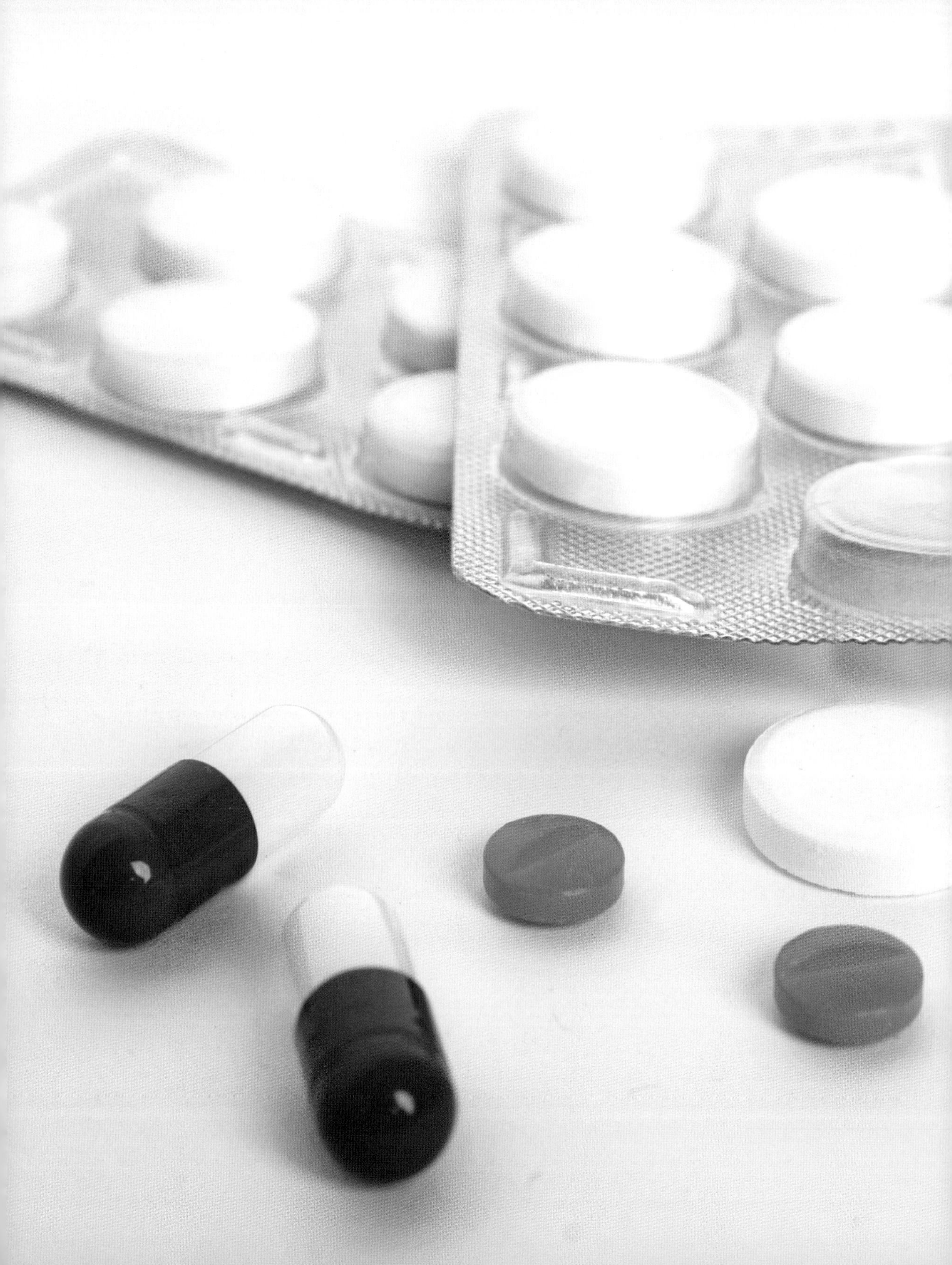

Review your medication on a regular basis to ensure that it is having the right effects on your body

Try this

- draw up a Medicine Record Chart (see page 157) and show the chart to your doctor on your next visit
- ask your doctor to review what you are currently taking and to consider whether there might be any interactions. Are all the medications necessary?
- revise your list once you and your doctor decide on what changes to make
- keep the list with you to review on a regular basis, both with your pharmacist and your doctor
- know which medications will give you adverse side effects, and think about how you can reduce the impact
- tie these ideas into your daily routine.

Sleep without pills

Research has shown that taking sleeping tablets over a long period of time is strongly linked to falls. It is best to avoid taking these sorts of pills if you can. If you take them for a long time, they can make you drowsy and confused during the day, giving you the sense of having a kind of hangover. If you do take them regularly, talk to your doctor about whether you can reduce the dosage.

There can be many reasons why you might be experiencing sleep disturbance. They can relate to

meet Luisa Luisa had a pendant made of opal with a little clasp. When she went out to lunch, she would pride herself on bringing out her pendant, undoing the clasp and taking out her lunchtime medication. It was a great way of remembering to take her pills.

anxiety, inactivity, medications, caffeine, being overweight, or respiratory or cardiac problems. Discuss this with your doctor if you think any of these reasons may be affecting your sleep patterns.

There are alternative strategies to cope with sleep problems and to help you avoid taking sleeping tablets. The following suggestions have been shown to be effective:

- go to bed when you are ready to sleep
- go to bed half an hour later than your usual time
- have a bedtime ritual—do the same thing each night
- avoid coffee and other drinks and foods with stimulants after 4 pm
- have regular exercise
- if you cannot sleep at night, then read or do some quiet activity. This works best if you don't stay in bed. Get up if you can, if it's not too cold
- avoid daytime naps
- keep the bedroom just for sleeping—and sexual activity
- keep clock faces turned away and try not to check the time when you wake during the night
- have a special "worry time" before you sleep so that you clear your head of problems before you go to sleep
- have enough daylight during the day—natural light helps with sleep/night cycles
- try relaxation or other special ways to help you sleep. Your library may have relaxation tapes you can borrow
- try not to worry about not sleeping.

Can you add to the list? What works for you?

If you have trouble sleeping, try doing some relaxation techniques before you go to bed

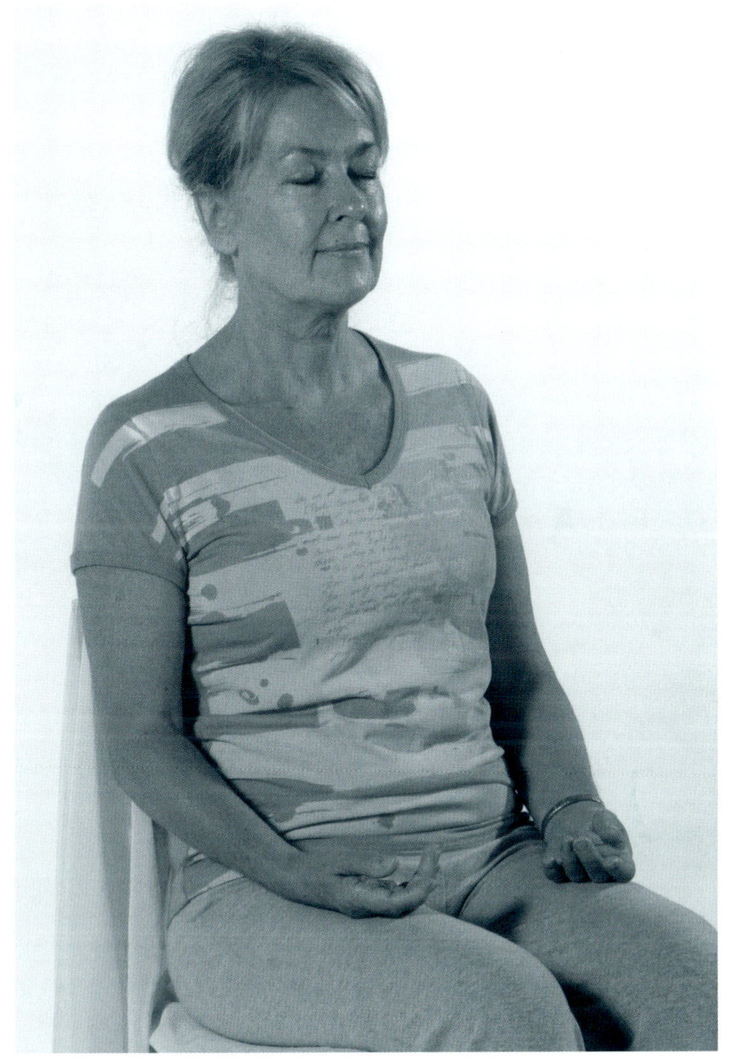

meet Jan After Jan had prepared her medication record, she was convinced many of her falls were related to her sleeping tablets. She talked to her doctor and he cut the dosage. This was really difficult to do as she believed she had come to rely on them and never thought there could be other options to help. She started to exercise more and made sure she got some good periods of sunlight during the day. She found going to bed an hour later particularly helpful.

CHAPTER 19

postural dizziness

Postural dizziness is defined as dizziness that occurs after you stand up. The sensation is described as feeling dizzy, faint, light-headed or woozy. While in some circumstances it can be related to poor balance and muscle strength, to medication or to drowsiness, postural dizziness is usually quite distinct.

Just as many people do not realise there are many ways to reduce the risk of falling, so too dizziness is too often accepted as an inevitable part of ageing. This attitude prevent people from finding out what can be done to recover from and to manage their dizziness.

Some of the reasons for postural dizziness can be inner-ear (vestibular) imbalance, visual problems or problems with the blood flow to and within the brain. Clearly these can pose significant problems, and not just in relation to falls. If you have persistent dizziness, see your doctor. They should be able to help you reduce the causes of your dizziness.

Tips for managing your dizziness

Here are some examples of how, with the help of medical professionals, you can manage your dizziness:

- undertake a medication review. Your medicines might be conflicting or overly strong, creating unnecessary side effects. Make sure your doctor knows about your dizziness when you do this so that they know what they are looking for

- have regular check-ups for your vision. This will make it easier to know where your dizziness is coming from, and what can be done about it
- ask for a referral to a neurologist or an ear, nose and throat specialist
- a physiotherapist or balance clinic can diagnose specific balance conditions related to the vestibular system. They can prescribe exercises that are very effective for these conditions.
- people with Parkinson's disease will benefit from a specialty Parkinson's group, if available, which will teach specific techniques for enhancing your mobility. This may also help with motivation to continue home exercises.

Dizziness is too often accepted as an inevitable part of ageing.

In addition, there are some more basic strategies you can use to manage postural dizziness yourself:

- implement safe habits that protect you from the risk of falling because of dizziness—stand up slowly, pause for a moment when you are on your feet and then make sure you are feeling steady before you move on
- purchase and wear supportive footwear. This will make it easier to feel surfaces such as step edges underneath you. The soles should not be too thick so they allow sensory feedback on the bottom of your feet
- use a cane or walking stick when you are outside. While using a cane will certainly help, it is better to investigate causes of the dizziness, and to improve your strength and balance as first options.

CHAPTER 20

benefits of vitamin D and calcium

It's well known that calcium is important for keeping your bones healthy and strong. Less known, however, is the importance of vitamin D. This vitamin helps your body absorb and use calcium, thereby keeping your bones and muscles strong. This in turn provides some protection from injury if you fall.

Vitamin D improves bone density and is high on the list of current recommendations to reduce osteoporosis. Vitamin D supplements combined with a diet rich in calcium have been proven to reduce the possibility of hip fracture from a fall. So build up your intake. The recommended daily intake of calcium for men older than 65 years is 800 mg per day and for women 1000 mg per day. Calcium is found in milk, yoghurt, hard cheeses and buttermilk. A glass of milk contains about 300–400 mg of calcium and a cube of cheese, about 200 mg. If you can't drink milk, try some soy products, fortified breads and/or orange juice.

Vitamin D sources

Vitamin D can be obtained from some food sources but these food types are not usually in our diet or not present in sufficient quantities. They include fish (especially salmon, tuna, sardines), cod liver oil and lambs fry (liver). We just can't rely on getting enough vitamin D from food. The easiest way to get vitamin D is by being in the sun. Vitamin D is formed in the skin by the action of ultraviolet B rays, which come from direct sunshine. Once made, vitamin D ends up being broken down and delivered to our muscles and bones, where, among other things, it helps to absorb calcium.

A little sunshine goes a long way

> The easiest way to get vitamin D is by being in the sun.

In the Southern Hemisphere, we often hear messages from the Cancer Council telling us to stay out of the sun, and for good reason. However, the kind of exposure required to get enough Vitamin D is not a lot. You just need some sun exposure on your arms for 8 to 10 minutes in summer and 20 minutes a day in winter. Sunshine has other positive benefits, not least of all a general feeling of wellbeing.

You don't need to go out in the sun during the hottest part of the day. You can even break the 20 minutes into 10-minute sections morning and afternoon. Studies have shown that 20 minutes a day, three times a week, will maintain adequate levels for many people.

Your doctor can test your level of vitamin D through a simple blood test. If necessary, they can recommend supplements to get your supply up to normal levels. To have the greatest effect, vitamin D needs to be absorbed on a regular basis, but you can get some help boosting it up to a healthy level or during winter months.

meet Andrew Andrew was a member of the senior computer club. He was an avid computer buff, being on the computer most days and only getting into his car to go to the shops. We asked people to record how much sunshine they were getting over a two-week period. He was surprised at how his lifestyle had changed and how little sun he now actually was getting. As a result, Andrew decided to walk to the shops more often so that he could benefit from the sunlight and get a healthy dose of vitamin D.

exercise record chart

3 Tick when I have done my exercises			
Week starting			
EXERCISES	**Day 1**	**Day 2**	**Day 3**
Balance Exercises			
Heel-toe standing			
Heel-toe walking			
Finding your toppling point			
Heel walking			
Sideways walk			
Strength exercises			
Sit-to-stand slowly			
Straight-leg raise			
Hip-strengthening side raise			
Calf raise			
Other exercises			

- Choose any three days of the week for your exercises but have a rest day between each one.
- Keep one of these charts every week for 7 to 12 weeks
- Keep upgrading to the next level as soon as you have mastered the balance exercise or find the weight not so hard to lift.

medicine record chart

Name:		Allergies:		Doctor's name and number:
Date prescribed	Medicine name	What it's for	Dose and how often	Special instructions/time of day (e.g. 1 hour before meals)

contacts and resources

If you would like to find out more on some of the areas covered in *Staying Power*, use the following information. Log on to the websites for quick access, or phone for details of what the various services have on offer.

ACCESSIBLE PUBLIC TRANSPORT

A link to all Australian public transport websites:
http://www.busaustralia.com/links.html

NSW
http://www.131500.info/realtime/default.asp
http://www.sydneybuses.info/accessibility
http://www.cityrail.info/facilities/accessing.jsp
Ph: 131500

West Australia
http://www.transperth.wa.gov.au/Default.aspx?tabid=46
Transperth InfoLine Ph: 136213

Queensland
http://www.translink.com.au/AccessibleTransport

For special assistance to travel with Citytrain:
Passenger Services Ph: (07) 3606 5555
or Telephone Typewriter Services,
Ph: (07) 3606 5800

QR Citytrain has introduced a SMS text messaging service for people with a disability. For more information, go to www.citytrain.com.au

Transport Access Guide
Ph: (07) 3253 0532
Email: trans@stjohnqld.asn.au

South Australia
http://www.adelaidemetro.com.au/general/accessible.html
Ph: (08) 8210 1000
or toll free on 1800 182 160

ACT
http://www.action.act.gov.au/accessible.cfm

Victoria
http://www.metlinkmelbourne.com.au/accessible/

The Met Information line has a TTY facility for passengers with hearing difficulties.
Ph: (03) 9619 2727

For advice on accessible travel nearest you:
Metlink telephone info line Ph: 131638

http://www.alphalink.com.au/~parkerp/meltrip/access.htm

THE STEPPING ON PROGRAM

Ask your local health centre if there is a Stepping On program near you. (see Carelink)

Stepping On manuals are available from:
Co-ordinates Therapy Services
PO Box 59
West Brunswick, Victoria, 3055
Ph: (03) 9380 1127
Email: jenny@therapybookshop.com
http://www.therapybookshop.com/

MORE INFORMATION ON BALANCE AND STRENGTH TRAINING

Accident Compensation Corporation *Otago Exercise Programme to Prevent Falls in Older Adults*, New Zealand, August 2003
http://www.acc.co.nz/injury-prevention/growing-and-living-safely

Fiatarone Singh MA *Exercise, Nutrition and the Older Woman: wellness for women over fifty*, CRC Press, London, 2000

USEFUL SERVICES

Commonwealth Carelink
Commonwealth Carelink provides free information about the care services available in your area, how to contact them, who is

eligible and whether there are any costs associated with the service
http://www.commcarelink.health.gov.au/
Ph: 1800 052 222

Home safety checklist for falls prevention
http://www.health.nsw.gov.au/health-public-affairs/mhcs/publications/5415.html

Independent Living Centres
These centres offer information on living independently in your own home and the community. They can help with modifications, aids and equipment, and will put you in touch with other services

NSW Ph: 1300 885 886
www.ilcnsw.asn.au

ACT Ph: (02) 6205 1900

QLD Ph: 1300 885 886 or (07) 3397 1224
www.ilcqld.org.au

SA Ph: 1800 800 523 (country areas) or (08) 8266 5260
www.ilc.asn.au

TAS Ph: 1300 651 166 or (03) 6334 5899
www.ilctas.asn.au

VIC Ph: 1800 686 533 (country areas) or (03) 9362 6111
http://deis.vic.gov.au

WA Ph: 1800 800 523 (country areas) or (08) 9381 0608
www.ilc.com.au

Low Vision Australia
Ph: 1800 331 000
www.visionaustralia.org.au

acknowledgments

We are grateful to Tom Swann for his editing and literary skills in helping us with our first draft, transforming Stepping On—our Falls Prevention program—into this book. Many thanks to Jayne Denshire and Limelight Press for their support and professionalism in making this book happen; and, to our family and friends who helped us along the way.

Thanks to the participants of Stepping On who contributed many stories and ideas, and inspired us to believe that falls prevention can make a difference. The Stepping On program was evaluated by a randomised trial, effectively reducing falls by 31 per cent. We would like to acknowledge the aid of the following people who contributed in varying ways to this research project: Bob Cumming, Rob Heard, Hal Kendig and Robyn Twible.

We also gratefully appreciate the expert contributions made by Ewa Borkowski, Shirley Carroll and Charles Butler in the early development of Stepping On. The initiative could not have been developed without the financial and in-kind support that enabled us to run our first programs. Special thanks to Valerie Joy at Leichhardt Council, Mercy Family Centre, Balmain Leagues Club and Burwood RSL.

Limelight Press would like to kindly thank Barry Bidwell, Kerry FitzGerald, Karen Gilroy and Margaret Williams for participating in the photos in this book.

index